THE VETERANS CHOICE PROGRAM (VCP)

ACCESS, IMPLEMENTATION AND IMPROVEMENTS

VETERANS: BENEFITS, ISSUES, POLICIES AND PROGRAMS

Additional books and e-books in this series can be found on Nova's website under the Series tab.

THE VETERANS CHOICE PROGRAM (VCP)

ACCESS, IMPLEMENTATION AND IMPROVEMENTS

MABEL PAGE
EDITOR

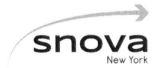

New York

NOTICE TO THE READER

Library of Congress Cataloging-in-Publication Data

ISBN: 978-1-53614-819-0

Published by Nova Science Publishers, Inc. † New York

CONTENTS

PREFACE

In response to concerns about access to medical care at many Department of Veterans Affairs (VA) hospitals and clinics across the country in spring 2014,1 Congress passed the Veterans Access, Choice, and Accountability Act of 2014 (VACAA, P.L. 113-146, as amended). On August 7, 2014, President Obama signed the bill into law. Among other things, the act establishes a new program that would allow the VA to authorize care for enrolled veterans through the Veterans Choice Program if they meet the eligibility requirements.

Chapter 1 - On August 7, 2014, President Obama signed the Veterans Access, Choice, and Accountability Act of 2014 (H.R. 3230; H.Rept. 113-564; P.L. 113-146). The Department of Veterans Affairs Expiring Authorities Act of 2014 (H.R. 5404; P.L. 113-175), the Consolidated and Further Continuing Appropriations Act, 2015 (H.R. 83; P.L. 113-235), the Construction Authorization and Choice Improvement Act (H.R. 2496; P.L. 114-19), and the Surface Transportation and Veterans Health Care Choice Improvement Act of 2015 (H.R. 3236; P.L. 114-41) made amendments to some provisions in P.L. 113-146. The act, as amended, makes a number of changes to programs and policies of the Veterans Health Administration (VHA) within the Department of Veterans Affairs (VA) that aim to increase access to care outside the VA health care system. Among other things, the act establishes a new program (the Veterans Choice Program) that would allow the VA to authorize care for enrolled veterans through the Veterans Choice Program if they meet the following eligibility requirements:

1. Attempts, or has attempted to schedule an appointment for the receipt of hospital care or medical services but is unable to schedule an appointment:
   within the wait-time goals of the VHA for the furnishing of care or services; or
   within a clinically appropriate period if such time frame is shorter than the wait-time goals of the VHA; or
2. Resides more than 40 miles (based on distance traveled):
   if seeking primary care, from a VA medical facility including a community-based outpatient clinic (CBOC) that is able to provide the care sought and provided by a full-time primary care physician; or
   if not seeking primary care, from any VA medical facility including a community-based outpatient clinic (CBOC); or
3. Resides in a state without a VA medical facility that provides (a) hospital care; (b) emergency medical services; and (c) surgical care, or more than 20 miles away from such a VA medical facility; or
4. Resides within 40 miles of a VA medical facility and is required to travel by air, boat, or ferry to access such a facility; or faces a travel burden based on geographical challenges; or inaccessible roads or hazardous weather; or a medical condition that would prevent the veteran from travelling; or any other factor as determined by the VHA.

This report offers an overview of the provisions in the law, which requires, among other things:

- increased collaboration between the VA and facilities operated by the Indian Health Service or the Native Hawaiian Health Care System and requiring increased funding for graduate medical education training at the VA;

- the extension of Project ARCH (Access Received Closer to Home) within specified Veterans Integrated Service Networks (VISNs) for veterans in highly rural areas who are enrolled in VA health care for an additional two years;
- several studies to examine a variety of issues pertaining to VA's health care delivery system, and to explore ideas on how best to reform the system;
- imposition of penalties on VA employees who knowingly falsify data on patient wait times or health care quality measures; and limitations on VA employee and bonuses.
-

Chapter 2 - Authorized under Section 101 of the Veterans Access, Choice, and Accountability Act of 2014 (VACAA), the Veterans Choice Program (VCP) is a new, temporary program that enables eligible veterans to receive medical care in the community. (P.L. 115-26 eliminated the August 7, 2017, expiration date for the VCP and allowed the program to continue until the initial $10 billion deposited in the Veterans Choice Fund was expended. The VA Choice and Quality Employment Act of 2017, P.L. 115-46, authorized and appropriated an additional $2.1 billion to continue the VCP until funds were expended, and when these funds were also nearing its end, Division D of P.L. 115-96 appropriated an additional $2.1 billion to continue the VCP until funds are expended.) It supplements several existing statutory authorities that allow the Veterans Health Administration (VHA) to provide health care services to veterans outside of the Department of Veterans Affairs (VA) facilities. Generally, all medical care and services (including inpatient, outpatient, pharmacy, and ancillary services) are provided through the VCP—institutional long-term care and emergency care in non-VA facilities are excluded from the VCP and are provided under different authorities. The VCP is not a health insurance plan for veterans, nor does it guarantee health care coverage to all veterans.

Eligibility and Choice of Care. Veterans must be enrolled in the VA health care system to request health services under the VCP. A veteran may request a VA community care consult/referral, or his or her VA provider may submit a VA community care consult/referral to the VA Care Coordination staff within the VA.

Veterans may become eligible for the VCP in one of four ways. First, a veteran is informed by a local VA medical facility that an appointment cannot be scheduled within 30 days of the clinically determined date requested by his or her VA doctor *or* within 30 days of the date requested by the veteran (this category also includes care not offered at a veterans' primary VA facility and a referral cannot be made to another VA medical facility or other federal facility). Second, the veteran lives 40 miles or more from a VA medical facility that has a full-time primary care physician. Third, the veteran lives 40 miles or less (not residing in Guam, America Samoa, or the Republic of the Philippines) *and* either travels by air, boat, or ferry to seek care from his or her local facility *or* incurs a traveling burden of a medical condition, geographic challenge, or an environmental factor. Fourth, the veteran resides 20 miles or more from a VA medical facility located in Alaska, Hawaii, New Hampshire (excluding those who live 20 miles from the White River Junction VAMC), or a U.S. territory, with the exception of Puerto Rico.

Once found eligible for care through the VCP, veterans may choose to receive care from a VA provider *or* from an eligible VA community care provider (VCP provider). VCP providers are federally-qualified health centers, Department of Defense (DOD) facilities, or Indian Health Service facilities, and hospitals, physicians, and nonphysician practitioners or entities participating in the Medicare or Medicaid program, among others. A veteran has the choice to switch between a VA provider and VCP provider at any time.

Program Administration and Provider Participation. The VCP is administered by two third-party administrators (TPAs): Health Net and TriWest. Generally, Health Net and TriWest manage veterans' appointments, counseling services, card distributions, and a call center. The TPAs contract directly with the VA. Then, Health Net or TriWest will contract with eligible non-VA community care providers interested on participating in the VCP. At the end of September 2018, the VA has announced that it would end its contract with Health Net as a TPA because of low patient volume, customer service issues and late payments to community providers in its network. It is anticipated that TriWest would continue to be a TPA for the areas they manage.

Payments. Generally, a veteran's out-of-pocket costs under the VCP are equal to VHA out-of-pocket costs. Veterans do not pay any copayments at the time of their medical appointments. Copayment rates are determined by the VA after services are furnished. Enactment of P.L. 115-26 on April 19, 2017, allowed VA to become the primary payer when certain veterans with other health insurance (OHI) receive care for nonservice-connected conditions under VCP—veterans would not have to pay a copayment under their OHI anymore. The VA would coordinate with a veteran's OHI and bill for any copayments that the veteran would be responsible for similar to what they would have paid had they received care within a VA medical facility. Participating community providers are reimbursed by their respective TPA, and VA pays the TPAs.

Chapter 3 - Congress created the Choice Program in 2014 to address longstanding challenges with veterans' access to care at VHA medical facilities. The Joint Explanatory Statement for the Consolidated Appropriations Act, 2016 included provisions for GAO to review veterans' access to care through the Choice Program.

This report examines for Choice Program care (1) VA's appointment scheduling process, (2) the timeliness of appointments and the information VHA uses to monitor veterans' access; and (3) the factors that have adversely affected veterans' access and the steps VA and VHA have taken to address them for VA's future community care program.

GAO reviewed applicable laws and regulations, VA's TPA contracts, and relevant VHA policies and guidance. Absent reliable national data, GAO also selected 6 of 170 VAMCs (selected for variation in geographic location and the TPAs that served them) and manually reviewed a random, non-generalizable sample of 196 Choice Program authorizations. The authorizations were created for veterans who were referred to the program between January and April of 2016, the most recent period for which data were available when GAO began its review. The sample of authorizations included 55 for routine care, 53 for urgent care, and 88 that the TPAs returned without scheduling appointments. GAO also obtained the results of VHA's non-generalizable analysis of wait times for a nationwide sample of about 5,000 Choice Program authorizations that were created for selected services between July and September of 2016.

Chapter 4 - Questions have been raised about the lack of timeliness of TPAs' payments to community providers under the Choice Program and how this may affect the willingness of providers to participate in the program as well as in the forthcoming Veterans Community Care Program. You asked GAO to review issues related to the timeliness of TPAs' payments to community providers under the Choice Program.

This chapter examines, among other things, (1) the length of time TPAs have taken to pay community providers' claims and factors affecting timeliness of payments, and (2) actions taken by VA and the TPAs to reduce the length of time TPAs take to pay community providers for Choice Program claims.

GAO reviewed TPA data on the length of time taken to pay community provider claims from November 2014 through June 2018, the most recent data available at the time of GAO's review. GAO also reviewed documentation, such as the contracts between VA and its TPAs, and interviewed VA and TPA officials. In addition, GAO interviewed a non-generalizable sample of 15 community providers, selected based on their large Choice Program claims volume, to learn about their experiences with payment timeliness.

In: The Veterans Choice Program (VCP)   ISBN: 978-1-53614-819-0
Editor: Mabel Page   © 2019 Nova Science Publishers, Inc.

Chapter 1

VETERANS ACCESS, CHOICE, AND ACCOUNTABILITY ACT OF 2014 (H.R. 3230; P.L. 113-146)*

Sidath Viranga Panangala, Maeve P. Carey, Cassandria Dortch and Elayne J. Heisler

SUMMARY

On August 7, 2014, President Obama signed the Veterans Access, Choice, and Accountability Act of 2014 (H.R. 3230; H.Rept. 113-564; P.L. 113-146). The Department of Veterans Affairs Expiring Authorities Act of 2014 (H.R. 5404; P.L. 113-175), the Consolidated and Further Continuing Appropriations Act, 2015 (H.R. 83; P.L. 113-235), the Construction Authorization and Choice Improvement Act (H.R. 2496; P.L. 114-19), and the Surface Transportation and Veterans Health Care Choice Improvement Act of 2015 (H.R. 3236; P.L. 114-41) made amendments to some provisions in P.L. 113-146. The act, as amended, makes a number of changes to programs and policies of the Veterans

---

* This is an edited, reformatted and augmented version of Congressional Research Service, Publication No. R43704, dated August 27, 2015.

Health Administration (VHA) within the Department of Veterans Affairs (VA) that aim to increase access to care outside the VA health care system. Among other things, the act establishes a new program (the Veterans Choice Program) that would allow the VA to authorize care for enrolled veterans through the Veterans Choice Program if they meet the following eligibility requirements:

1. Attempts, or has attempted to schedule an appointment for the receipt of hospital care or medical services but is unable to schedule an appointment: within the wait-time goals of the VHA for the furnishing of care or services; or
   within a clinically appropriate period if such time frame is shorter than the wait-time goals of the VHA; or
2. Resides more than 40 miles (based on distance traveled):
   if seeking primary care, from a VA medical facility including a community-based outpatient clinic (CBOC) that is able to provide the care sought and provided by a full-time primary care physician; or
   if not seeking primary care, from any VA medical facility including a community-based outpatient clinic (CBOC); or
3. Resides in a state without a VA medical facility that provides (a) hospital care; (b) emergency medical services; and (c) surgical care, or more than 20 miles away from such a VA medical facility; or
4. Resides within 40 miles of a VA medical facility and is required to travel by air, boat, or ferry to access such a facility; or faces a travel burden based on geographical challenges; or inaccessible roads or hazardous weather; or a medical condition that would prevent the veteran from travelling; or any other factor as determined by the VHA.

This chapter offers an overview of the provisions in the law, which requires, among other things:

- increased collaboration between the VA and facilities operated by the Indian Health Service or the Native Hawaiian Health Care System and requiring increased funding for graduate medical education training at the VA;
- the extension of Project ARCH (Access Received Closer to Home) within specified Veterans Integrated Service Networks (VISNs) for

veterans in highly rural areas who are enrolled in VA health care for an additional two years;

- several studies to examine a variety of issues pertaining to VA's health care delivery system, and to explore ideas on how best to reform the system;
- imposition of penalties on VA employees who knowingly falsify data on patient wait times or health care quality measures; and limitations on VA employee and bonuses.

INTRODUCTION

This chapter uses a number of acronyms, which are listed below.

CBO   Congressional Budget Office; also Chief Business Office of the Veterans Health Administration
CBOC   Community Based Outpatient Clinic
DOD   Department of Defense
FQHCs   Federally Qualified Health Centers
GAO   Government Accountability Office
HHS   Department of Health and Human Services
IHS   Indian Health Service
MST   Military Sexual Trauma
NVCC   Non-VA Care Coordination Project
ARCH   Access Received Closer to Home
U.S.C.   United States Code
VA   Department of Veterans Affairs
VAMC   VA Medical Center
VHA   Veterans Health Administration
VISNs   Veterans Integrated Service Networks

In April 2014, Congress became aware of issues pertaining to delays in patient care and patient wait time manipulation at various Department of

Veterans Affairs (VA) health care system facilities.[1] In response to these issues, in August 2014 Congress passed the Veterans Access, Choice, and Accountability Act of 2014 (P.L. 113-146). At the heart of this legislation is a temporary new program known as the "Veterans Choice Program," intended to increase eligible veterans' access to care through eligible non-VA providers and facilities. In addition, P.L. 113- 146, as amended, provides additional funding to improve VA's physical infrastructure and to hire physicians and other medical professionals, including nurses, mental health professionals, and social workers. Lastly, among other things, the Veterans Access, Choice, and Accountability Act of 2014 requires the VA to enter into one or more contracts with a private sector entity or entities for an independent assessment in order to comprehensively examine the VA's ability to deliver high-quality health care to veterans now and into the future. As discussed in the next section, the act (P.L. 113-146) has been amended several times since it was enacted on August 7, 2014. This chapter begins with a brief overview of the legislative history that lead up to the enactment of the Veterans Access, Choice, and Accountability Act of 2014, and subsequent amendments to the act.

BRIEF LEGISLATIVE HISTORY

In an attempt to address delays in patient care provided by the VA health care system and to provide veterans with timely access to care, among other things, the Senate and House introduced and passed several measures in May and June of 2014. Initially, on June 9, 2014, the Veterans' Access to Care through Choice, Accountability, and Transparency Act of 2014 (S. 2450) was introduced in the Senate, and the Veteran Access to Care Act of 2014 (H.R. 4810) was introduced in the House. The House passed its measure on June 10, but the Senate chose to act on its proposal by substituting the text of S. 2450 for that of H.R. 3230, a measure previously received from the

---

[1] U.S. Congress, House Committee on Veterans' Affairs, *A Continued Assessment of Delays in VA Medical Care and Preventable Veteran Deaths'*, 113th Cong., 2nd sess., April 9, 2014.

House.[2] The House then amended the Senate substitute for H.R. 3230 by substituting the text of H.R. 4810 and also that of the Department of Veterans Affairs Management Accountability Act of 2014 (H.R. 4031), a measure it had previously passed on May 21. This action enabled the two chambers to proceed to conference on their respective versions of H.R. 3230.

On July 28, the Co-Chairmen of the Conference Committee, Senator Bernie Sanders and Representative Jeff Miller, announced that an agreement had been reached, and reported the measure. The conferees voted on the conference report (H.Rept. 113-564) on the same day.[3] The full House passed the Veterans Access, Choice, and Accountability Act of 2014 (H.R. 3230; H.Rept. 113-564) on July 30, and the Senate passed the conference measure on July 31. President Barack Obama signed the Veterans Access, Choice, and Accountability Act of 2014 into law (P.L. 113-146) on August 7, 2014.[4]

On September 26, 2014, the Department of Veterans Affairs Expiring Authorities Act of 2014 (H.R. 5404; P.L. 113-175) was signed into law. Sections 408 and 409 of P.L. 113-175 made minor amendments to Sections 101, 102, 104, 105, 204, 206, 207, 301, 302, and 702 of the Veterans Access, Choice, and Accountability Act of 2014. On December 16, 2014, President Barack Obama signed into law the Consolidated and Further Continuing Appropriations Act, 2015 (H.R. 83; P.L. 113-235). Division I of this act contained the Military Construction and Veterans Affairs, and Related Agencies Appropriations Act, 2015. Section 242 of this act amended Section 101 of the Veterans Access, Choice, and Accountability Act of 2014. On May 22, 2015, the Construction Authorization and Choice Improvement Act (H.R. 2496; P.L. 114-19) was enacted into law. Section

---

[2] The Senate took this course of action because S. 2450 contained appropriations, which the House traditionally insists must be enacted in a measure it has originated. H.R. 3230 was available for this purpose because Congress had acted in other legislation on issues that H.R. 3230 originally addressed.

[3] "Conference Report on H.R. 3230," *Congressional Record*, daily edition, vol.160 (July 28, 2014), pp. H6953-H6974; and U.S. Congress, Committee of Conference, *Veterans Access, Choice, and Accountability Act of 2014*, Report to Accompany H.R. 3230, 113th Cong., 2nd sess., July 28, 2014, H.Rept. 113-564 (Washington: GPO, 2013), pp. 3-81.

[4] While some provisions took effect on that same date, other provisions such as the new authority that would allow veterans to seek care from non-VA health care providers will not take effect until implementing regulations are issued.

3 of this act amended Section 101(b)(2)of the Veterans Access, Choice, and Accountability Act of 2014, as amended. Lastly, on July 31, 2015, the Surface Transportation and Veterans Health Care Choice Improvement Act of 2015 (H.R. 3236; P.L. 114-41) was enacted into law. Title IV of this act contained the VA Budget and Choice Improvement Act. Sections 4004 and 4005 of this act amended and modified Sections 101 and 802 of the Veterans Access, Choice, and Accountability Act of 2014. The summary of selected provisions of the Veterans Access, Choice, and Accountability Act of 2014 (P.L. 113-146) provided in this report incorporates these amendments made by P.L. 113-175, P.L. 113-235, P.L. 114-19, and P.L. 114- 41.

PROVISIONS IN THE VETERANS ACCESS, CHOICE, AND ACCOUNTABILITY ACT OF 2014

The rest of this chapter provides a summary of selected provisions in the Veterans Access, Choice, and Accountability Act of 2014 (P.L. 113-146)— as amended by the Department of Veterans Affairs Expiring Authorities Act of 2014 (H.R. 5404; P.L. 113-175); the Consolidated and Further Continuing Appropriations Act, 2015 (H.R. 83; P.L. 113-235); the Construction Authorization and Choice Improvement Act (H.R. 2496; P.L. 114-19); and the Surface Transportation and Veterans Health Care Choice Improvement Act of 2015 (H.R. 3236; P.L. 114-41)—by title and section. It does not attempt to analyze each of the provisions in the act in depth, but provides brief outlines of the matters addressed. The *Appendix* provides a table showing the numerous implementing and reporting deadlines required by P.L. 113-146 as amended by P.L. 113-175. Throughout this chapter, unless otherwise stated, the "Secretary" means the Secretary of Veterans Affairs, and the "VA" means the same. In addition, "this section" refers to matters addressed under that specific section of the act.

Sec. 1. Short Title

This section provides the title of the bill as the "Veterans Access, Choice, and Accountability Act of 2014."

Sec. 2. Definitions

This section provides definitions of the terms used for the purposes of this act. These definitions refer to current law definitions provided in Title 38 U.S.C. for the terms "facilities of the Department," "hospital care," and "medical services."[5]

TITLE I: IMPROVEMENT OF ACCESS TO CARE FROM NON-DEPARTMENT OF VETERANS AFFAIRS PROVIDERS

At the core of this title is a new *temporary* program (the Veterans Choice Program) to provide hospital care and medical services to certain eligible veterans in non-VA facilities or through non-VA providers. The VA has 90 days from the date of enactment (i.e., November 5, 2014) to issue interim final regulations to implement major provisions of Section 101.[6]

---

[5] 38 U.S.C. §1701. Under current law, the term "facilities of the Department" means facilities over which the Secretary has direct jurisdiction; other VA- contracted government facilities; and public or private facilities at which the Secretary provides recreational activities for patients receiving VA care. The terms "hospital care" and "medical services" have the meanings given such terms by 38 U.S.C. §1701(5) and §1701(6).

[6] For a discussion of implementation issues of the Veterans Choice Program, see CRS In Focus IF10224, *Implementation of the Veterans Choice Program (VCP)*, by Sidath Viranga Panangala.

Sec. 101. Availability of Hospital Care and Medical Services through the Use of Non-VA Entities

Eligibility

This section requires the VA to authorize non-VA care to veterans who are enrolled in the VA health care system, including a veteran enrolled in the VA health care system who has not received hospital care or medical services from the VA and has contacted the VA seeking an initial appointment for the receipt of such care or services; [7]

If a veteran is enrolled in the VA health system, then veterans are eligible for Veterans Choice Program authorization if they meet one of the following four criteria:

(A) attempts, or has attempted to schedule an appointment for the receipt of hospital care or medical services but is unable to schedule an appointment.

> (I)   within the wait-time goals of the VHA for the furnishing of care or services; or
> (II) within a clinically appropriate period if such time frame is shorter than the wait-time goals of the VHA;[8]

or

> (B) resides more than 40 miles (based on distance traveled),[9]
> (I)   if seeking primary care, from a VA medical facility including a community-based outpatient clinic (CBOC) that is able to provide

---

[7] Prior to the passage of the Surface Transportation and Veterans Health Care Choice Improvement Act of 2015 (H.R. 3236; P.L. 114-41), veterans had to have been enrolled in the VA health care system as of August 1, 2014, or have to have served in a combat-theater and discharged or released from active duty during a five-year period prior to the enrollment date. With the enactment of P.L. 114-41, these criteria no longer applies.

[8] As amended by the Surface Transportation and Veterans Health Care Choice Improvement Act of 2015 (H.R. 3236; P.L. 114-41).

[9] As amended by the Construction Authorization and Choice Improvement Act (H.R. 2496; P.L. 114-19). The VA would generally use driving distance when measuring the distance traveled from a veteran's place of residence to the nearest VA medical facility, instead of a geodesic or straight-line distance measurement. The VA will calculate a veteran's driving distance using geographic information system (GIS) software.

the care sought and provided by a full-time primary care physician;[10] or

(II) if not seeking primary care, from any VA medical facility including a community-based outpatient clinic (CBOC); [11]

or

(C) resides in a state without a VA medical facility that provides (I) hospital care, and (II) emergency medical services, and (III) surgical care rated by the Secretary as having a surgical complexity standard; *and* more than 20 miles from a VA medical facility that provides hospital care; and (II) emergency medical services; and (III) surgical care rated by the Secretary as having a surgical complexity standard;[12]

---

[10] As amended by the Surface Transportation and Veterans Health Care Choice Improvement Act of 2015 (H.R. 3236; P.L. 114-41). A veteran would be eligible for *primary care* through the Veterans Choice Program if the veteran *lives less than* 40 miles (as calculated based on distance traveled) from a VA medical facility, including a CBOC, if that facility is not able to provide the *primary care* sought by the veteran and cannot be provided by a full-time primary care physician. It should be noted that the VA is in the process of modifying its interim final rules (**Department of Veterans Affairs**, " Interim Final Rule - Expanded Access to Non-VA Care through the Veterans Choice Program," 79 *Federal Register* 65571 - 65587, November 5, 2014), and may through rulemaking, define how these latest eligibility criteria will be implemented.

[11] For a veteran *not seeking primary care*, the veteran would be eligible for care through the Veterans Choice Program system if the veteran lives more than 40 miles (as calculated based on distance traveled) from any VA medical facility. It should be noted that the VA is in the process of modifying its interim final rules (Department of Veterans Affairs, " Interim Final Rule - Expanded Access to Non-VA Care through the Veterans Choice Program," 79 *Federal Register* 65571 - 65587, November 5, 2014), and may through rulemaking, define how these latest eligibility criteria will be implemented.

[12] VA has assigned each of its medical centers an inpatient "surgical complexity" level—complex, intermediate or standard. Hospitals assigned a "complex" rating require special facilities, equipment and staff for difficult operations, such as cardiac surgery and craniotomies. Those with an "intermediate" rating may perform less complex surgeries, such as partial colon removal and complete joint replacement. Those with a "standard" rating may perform inpatient surgeries, such as hernia repair and ear, nose, and throat (ENT) surgeries. These measures were implemented May 7, 2010. If a VA hospital cannot provide a certain type of therapy or treatment to a patient, it will transfer the veteran to a VA facility that has these programs.

or

    (D) resides in a location, (*not including* a location in Guam, American Samoa or the Republic of the Philippines), that is 40 miles or less from a VA medical facility, including a CBOC;

and

    (1) is required to travel by air, boat, or ferry to reach each VA medical facility, including a CBOC, that is 40 miles or less from the veteran's residence

or

    (1) resides in a location, (*not including* a location in Guam, American Samoa, or the Republic of the Philippines), that is 40 miles or less from a VA medical facility, including a CBOC, and faces an unusual or excessive burden in accessing such a VA medical facility due to geographical challenges; *or* environmental factors, such as roads that are not accessible to the public, because of traffic, or hazardous weather; *or* a medical condition that impacts the veteran's ability to travel; or other factors, as determined by the VA.[13]

Choice of Provider

Eligible veterans authorized to receive care under this section could choose to receive care through any of the following non-VA entities or providers: Medicare providers, including any physician furnishing services

---

[13] As amended by the Construction Authorization and Choice Improvement Act (H.R. 2496; P.L. 114-19).

under such program;[14] FQHCs;[15] DOD medical facilities; IHS facilities; and other health care providers that meets criteria established by the Secretary.[16]

Coordination of Care with Non-VA Entities

This section requires the VA to use the Non-VA Care Coordination (NVCC) program to coordinate care of eligible veterans with non-VA providers. It also requires the VA to ensure that appointments are scheduled within the wait-time goals of the VA.[17]

Authorization of Care by the VA

This section requires the VA to authorize care to eligible veterans. It also allows the veteran to elect whether he or she wants to receive care from non-VA entities. If the veteran does not elect to receive care from non-VA entities, the veteran could be provided with an appointment that exceeds the wait-time goals of the VA,[18] or the veteran will be placed on an electronic waiting list—which may be viewed by the veteran—maintained by the VA for an appointment for hospital care or medical services. If the veteran chooses to be seen by non-VA entities, the VA is required to authorize such care or services to the eligible veteran for a period of time specified by the Secretary; and notify the eligible veteran by electronic communication or in writing, describing the care or services that the veteran is eligible to receive.

---

[14] Title XIII of the Social Security Act ("Medicare") 42 U.S.C. §1395 et seq. Medicare providers include physicians and psychologists, as well as patient care institutions such as hospitals, critical access hospitals, hospices, nursing homes, and home health agencies. See, http://www.cms.gov/Medicare/Provider-Enrollment-and-Certification/Certificationand Complianc/index.html.

[15] These include FQHC Look-Alike facilities. For more details, see CRS Report R42433, *Federal Health Centers*, by Elayne J. Heisler.

[16] As amended by the Surface Transportation and Veterans Health Care Choice Improvement Act of 2015 (H.R. 3236; P.L. 114-41).

[17] NVCC is an internal program to improve referral management practices. It was formerly known as "Fee Basis," "Purchased Care," or "Non-VA Care."

[18] As amended by Department of Veterans Affairs Expiring Authorities Act of 2014 (P.L. 113-175). As required by law, wait-time goals of the VA were published on October 17, 2014. See Department of Veterans Affairs, "Wait-Time Goals of the Department for the Veterans Choice Program," 79 *Federal Register* 62519-62520, October 17, 2014.

Electronic Waiting List

This section requires the VA to maintain an electronic waiting list and allow each eligible veteran access to it either through the www.myhealth.va.gov or any successor website (or other digital channel).[19] The veteran could use the electronic waiting list to determine the average length of time an individual spends on the waiting list at each specific VA medical facility. The veteran could use this information to decide if they want to seek care from a non-VA entity.

Care and Services through Agreements

This section requires the VA to enter into agreements for furnishing care and services to eligible veterans with the following entities: Medicare providers, including any physician furnishing services under such program;[20] FQHCs;[21] DOD medical facilities; IHS facilities; and other health care providers that meets criteria established by the Secretary.[22] This section defines the term "agreement" to include contracts, inter-governmental agreements, and provider agreements, as appropriate. Furthermore, this section stipulates that an agreement entered for furnishing care and services to eligible veterans cannot be treated as a federal contract for the acquisition of goods or services. This section also requires the Secretary to the maximum extent practicable to furnish care and services to eligible veterans using existing contracts or other processes available at VAMCs prior to entering into new agreements.[23]

---

[19] As amended by the Department of Veterans Affairs Expiring Authorities Act of 2014 (P.L. 113-175).

[20] Title XIII of the Social Security Act ("Medicare") 42 U.S.C. §1395 et seq. Medicare providers include physicians and psychologists, as well as patient care institutions such as hospitals, critical access hospitals, hospices, nursing homes, and home health agencies. See, http://www.cms.gov/Medicare/Provider-Enrollment-and-Certification/ CertificationandComplianc/index.html.

[21] These include FQHC Look-Alike facilities. For more details, see CRS Report R42433, *Federal Health Centers*, by Elayne J. Heisler.

[22] As amended by the Surface Transportation and Veterans Health Care Choice Improvement Act of 2015 (H.R. 3236; P.L. 114-41)

[23] As amended by the Department of Veterans Affairs Expiring Authorities Act of 2014 (P.L. 113-175).

Rates of Reimbursement

This section requires the Secretary to negotiate reimbursement rates for the furnishing of care and services with non-VA entities. Furthermore, this section places a limit on the reimbursement rate with several exceptions. In general, negotiated rates must be no more than the payment rate under the Medicare program under Title XVIII of the Social Security Act, set by the Centers for Medicare & Medicaid Services. However, the VA may negotiate a higher rate than the Medicare reimbursement rate if the provider is furnishing care or services to an eligible veteran who resides in a highly rural area (defined as an area located in a county that has fewer than seven individuals residing in that county per square mile). Furthermore, in the State of Alaska, VA will be able to reimburse providers under the VA Alaska Fee Schedule, and in states with an "All-Payer Model" agreement, VA will calculate Medicare payments based on payment rates under such All-Payer Model" agreements.[24] This section also exempts Medicare and Medicaid providers—during the period they are furnishing care to eligible veterans—from Federal Contract Compliance Programs of the Department of Labor that apply to federal contractors and subcontractors. Furthermore, this section stipulates that a non-VA health care entity may not collect an amount that is greater than the rate that was negotiated with the VA for care to eligible veterans. It also requires that the Secretary provide non-VA health care entities and providers with required information on policies and procedures with regard to billing, claims submission, and care authorization, among other things.

---

[24] As amended by the Consolidated and Further Continuing Appropriations Act, 2015 (P.L. 113-235). Maryland operates the nation's only all-payer hospital rate regulation system. Under Section 1814(b) (3) of the Social Security Act, the Centers for Medicare & Medicaid Services ("CMS") has exempted certain hospitals in Maryland from reimbursement under the national payment system and has allowed the state to set reimbursement rates payable by Medicare for applicable services that otherwise would be reimbursed under Medicare's Inpatient Prospective Payment System ("IPPS") and Outpatient Prospective Payment System ("OPPS"). On January 10, 2014, CMS and the State of Maryland jointly announced a new initiative to modernize Maryland's unique all-payer rate-setting system for hospital services. In the state of Maryland, VA will follow this reimbursement system.

VA as the Secondary Payer of Care

This section of the act stipulates that the VA will generally be the secondary payer[25] for eligible veterans receiving care for nonservice-connected disabilities or conditions from specified non-VA health care entities. It further stipulates that the VA will pay for care or services that are not covered by the veteran's health insurance plan at an amount not to exceed the Medicare rate or a negotiated rate. Furthermore, before receiving hospital care or medical services, an eligible veteran is required to provide the Secretary information on any insurance policy or contract that the veteran has. For those veterans who are only enrolled in Medicare, Medicaid, or TRICARE, the VA will be the primary payer for care and services for nonservice-connected disabilities or conditions.[26]

Veterans Choice Card

This section stipulates that not later than 90 days after enactment the VA is required to provide each enrolled veteran with a card known as a "Veterans Choice Card." Among other things, as specified, the following statement will be printed on the card: "This card is for qualifying medical care outside the Department of Veterans Affairs. Please call the Department of Veterans Affairs phone number specified on this card to ensure that treatment has been authorized." Furthermore, the act stipulates that the Secretary provide the eligible veteran with information clearly stating the circumstances under which the veteran may be eligible for care or services

Information on Availability of Care

This section requires the Secretary to provide information on non-VA care to veterans when they enroll in the VA health care system, when the veteran attempts to schedule an appointment for the receipt of hospital care or medical services from the VA but is unable to schedule an appointment within the current wait-time goals of the VHA for the delivery of such care

---

[25] A secondary payer is an insurance carrier or program that is secondary to the primary insurance carrier or program.

[26] VA will be a secondary payer in situations that the veteran has private coverage or other health care coverage that is not Medicare, Medicaid or TRICARE.

or services, and when the veteran becomes eligible for hospital care or medical services under this act.

Follow-Up Care

This section requires non-VA care authorizations to include a complete episode of care, including all specialty and ancillary services deemed necessary as part of an episode of recommended treatment.[27]

Credentials of Providers

This section of the act requires participating non-VA providers to maintain the same or similar credentials and licenses as required of VA health care providers, and to submit verification at least annually.

Copayments

This section of the act requires veterans who are authorized to receive non-VA care to pay applicable copayment just as they would be assessed a copayment if treatment was provided in a VA facility. The non-VA health care provider or entity that furnishes the care or service will be required to collect the copayment directly from the eligible veteran.

Health Care Claims Processing

This section requires the Secretary to establish an efficient nationwide system for processing and paying non-VA care bills or claims, and the Chief Business Office (CBO) of the VHA will oversee the implementation and maintenance of the claims processing system. Regulations implementing such a claims processing system are to be published no later than 90 days after enactment of this act.

---

[27] Prior to the passage of the Surface Transportation and Veterans Health Care Choice Improvement Act of 2015 (H.R. 3236; P.L. 114-41), authorization for care through the Veterans Choice Program was limited for a period of 60 days per episode of care. With the enactment of P.L. 114-41, this criterion no longer applies.

Medical Records

This section requires the VA to ensure that non-VA providers submit to the VA a copy of any medical record information related to the care and services provided to an eligible veteran for inclusion in the veteran's Computerized Patient Record System (CPRS) maintained by the VA. It further stipulates that to the greatest extent possible the medical records submitted by non-VA providers or entities should be in an electronic format.[28]

Tracking Missed Appointments

This section of the act requires the Secretary to implement a mechanism to track missed appointments authorized under this section for eligible veterans to ensure that the VA does not pay for such care or services that were not furnished to an eligible veteran.

Implementing Regulations

This section of the act requires the VA to prescribe and publish interim final regulations no later than 90 days after the date of the enactment on the implementation of the new program to provide eligible veterans with care in non-VA facilities.

Office of the Inspector General (OIG) Report

This section of the act requires the VA Inspector General to issue an audit of care report to the Secretary on the expanded non-VA care authority. The report is required to be submitted no later than 30 days after the Secretary determines that 75% of amounts deposited in the "Veterans Choice Fund" (see section on "Sec. 802. Veterans Choice Fund" later in this report) have been exhausted.

---

[28] As amended by the Department of Veterans Affairs Expiring Authorities Act of 2014 (P.L. 113-175).

End Date of the Expanded Authority for Non-VA Care

This section stipulates that the authority for the new expanded non-VA care program will end on a date when all the funds deposited in the "Veterans Choice Fund" (see section on "Sec. 802. Veterans Choice Fund" later in this chapter) are exhausted or on a date that is three years after the date of enactment, whichever comes first.

Reports to Congress

This section of the act requires the VA to submit reports to Congress on the expanded non-VA care authority. The Secretary is required to submit an interim report to Congress, not later than 90 days after the publication of interim final regulations. The interim report must include information on the number of eligible veterans and a description of the type of care and services furnished to eligible veterans. A final report is required no later than 30 days after the date on which the Secretary determines that 75% of the amounts deposited in the "Veterans Choice Fund" are exhausted. The final report must include, among other things, an assessment and recommendations regarding the continuation of non-VA care and services under the new expanded authority.

Filling Prescription Medications

This section specifies that VA's current practice of filling prescriptions of veterans at VA pharmacies and/or Consolidated Mail Order Pharmacies (CMOPs), and the policies that allow the VA to pay for prescribed drugs provided for certain eligible veterans, will continue without any changes.

Wait-Time Goals of the VHA

This section of the act defines "wait time goals of the Veterans Health Administration" as an appointment date that is not more than 30 days from the date that the veteran requested an appointment for care. If the Secretary notifies Congress no later than 60 days after enactment that the "wait-time goals of the Veterans Health Administration" are different than what is defined in this section, then the new wait time goals of the VHA will be the ones defined by the Secretary.[29]

Waiver of Certain Printing Requirements

This section allows the Secretary to print material related to the Veterans Choice Program other than through the Government Printing Office (GPO).[30]

Sec. 102. Enhancement of Collaboration between the VA and Indian Health Service

This section requires the Secretary (in consultation with the IHS Director) to conduct outreach to each medical facility operated by an Indian Tribe or Tribal Organization[31] to make these facilities aware that they can enter into agreements with the VA under which the VA will reimburse these facilities for care provided to IHS beneficiaries who are also VA-enrolled veterans. This section also requires the Secretary and the IHS director to jointly establish and implement performance metrics that examine whether the existing MOU between the VA and IHS—"Memorandum of

---

[29] On October 17, 2014, the Department of Veterans Affairs published a notice in the *Federal Register* announcing VA's report on the wait-time goals for purposes of the Veterans Choice Program. The report provides that the goals of the Veterans Health Administration are as follows: "Unless changed by further notice in the Federal Register, the term 'wait-time goals of the Veterans Health Administration' means not more than 30 days from either the date that an appointment is deemed clinically appropriate by a VA health care provider, or if no such clinical determination has been made, the date a Veteran prefers to be seen for hospital care or medical services. In the event a VA health care provider identifies a time range when care must be provided (e.g., within the next 2 months), VA will use the last clinically appropriate date for determining whether or not such care is timely. The Department anticipates that the Under Secretary for Health periodically will consider changes to the wait-time goals of the Veterans Health Administration as appropriate." See Department of Veterans Affairs, "Wait-Time Goals of the Department for the Veterans Choice Program," 79 *Federal Register* 62519-62520, October 17, 2014.

[30] As amended by the Department of Veterans Affairs Expiring Authorities Act of 2014 (P.L. 113-175). Section 501 of Title 44 of the United States Code requires that all printing for the executive departments and independent offices and establishments of the government be done through the Government Printing Office (GPO).

[31] For more information about the Indian Health Service, see CRS Report R43330, *The Indian Health Service (IHS): An Overview*, by Elayne J. Heisler.

Understanding" between the Department of Veterans Affairs (VA) and the Indian Health Service (IHS)—is effective at, among other things, increasing access, improving quality and care coordination, and determining whether health promotion and disease prevention services are funded and available to beneficiaries under both health care systems. The section further requires that the Secretary and the IHS Director submit a report to Congress on the (1) feasibility of including Urban Indian Organizations in the current VA-IHS reimbursement agreement, (2) feasibility of including the direct care costs of treating non-American Indian veterans in agreements between the VA and IHS facilities or medical facilities operated by an Indian Tribe or Tribal Organization, and (3) possible effects of an agreement between the IHS-VA agreement to provide care to veterans at IHS facilities on access to services by IHS-beneficiaries. This report is due no later than 180 days after enactment.[32]

Sec. 103. Enhancement of Collaboration between the VA and the Native Hawaiian Health Care System

This section requires the VA, in consultation with Papa Ola Lokahi and such other organizations involved in the delivery of health care to Native Hawaiians, to enter into contracts or agreements with Native Hawaiian health care systems, receiving funds from the Secretary of Health and Human Services (HHS), to reimburse such systems for direct care services provided to eligible veterans (as specified in the particular contract or agreement).

---

[32] As amended by the Department of Veterans Affairs Expiring Authorities Act of 2014 (P.L. 113-175).

Sec. 104. Reauthorization and Modification of Project ARCH (Access Received Closer to Home)

This section reauthorizes and modifies the pilot program known as Project ARCH, which was established under Section 403 of the Veterans' Mental Health and Other Care Improvements Act of 2008 (P.L. 110-387). The three-year pilot program was set to expire on August 29, 2014.[33] This section authorizes Project ARCH for two years from the date of enactment of the act. This section stipulates in law the pilot sites as: VISN 1; VISN 6; VISN 15; VISN 18; and VISN 19.[34] This section of the act further stipulates that the Secretary must ensure that medical appointments for those veterans eligible to participate in Project ARCH are scheduled not later than 5 days after the date on which the appointment is requested and occur no later than

---

[33] The Veterans' Mental Health and Other Care Improvements Act of 2008 (P.L. 110-387) was signed into law on October 10, 2008. Section 403 of this law required VA to conduct pilot programs during a three-year period to provide non-VA health care services through contractual arrangements to eligible veterans. This pilot program had an implementation date of 120 days after October 10, 2008. Soon after the law was enacted VA recognized that the pilot program could not be commenced in the 120 days of the law's enactment as required, and in March 2009, VA officials briefed House and Senate VA Committees on these implementation issues. The first challenge that VA shared with Congress was the statute's definition of highly rural. The statute uses driving distances to define a highly rural veteran whereas VA uses a Census Bureau definition and defines a highly rural veteran as a veteran who resides in a county with fewer than seven civilians per square mile. VA has developed its data systems based on the Census Bureau definition and uses these systems to identify highly rural veterans. The second challenge involved the term hardship which VA needs to define through regulations. The Caregiver and Veterans Omnibus Health Services Act of 2010 (P.L. 111-163) signed into law in May 2010 made technical corrections regarding hardship exception and the mileage standard. Those eligible to participate in Project ARCH include (1) veterans who are enrolled in the VA health care system as of the date of the commencement of the pilot program and meet the statutory definition of "covered Veterans", or (2) eligible but not enrolled Operation Enduring Freedom/Operation Iraqi Freedom/Operation New Dawn (OEF/OIF/OND) veterans who meet the statutory definition of "covered Veterans." Covered veterans are defined as those veterans residing in a Pilot VISN and are (1) more than 60 minutes away from the nearest VA health care facility providing primary care services, or (2) more than 120 minutes away from the nearest VA health care facility providing acute hospital care, or (3) more than 240 minutes away from the nearest VA health care facility providing tertiary care.

[34] The VA's health care system is organized into 21 geographically defined Veterans Integrated Service Networks (VISNs). VISN offices oversee VA healthcare facilities community based outpatient clinics, nursing homes, and Vet Centers throughout the country.

30 days after such date. This section allows the Secretary to use existing Project ARCH contracts or enter into new contracts.[35]

Sec. 105. Prompt Payment

This section states that it is the sense of Congress that the VA must comply with the Prompt Payment rule,[36] and requires VA to establish and implement a system to process and pay claims from non-VA providers for hospital care, medical services, and other health care services provided to eligible veterans. Furthermore, it requires the Government Accountability Office (GAO) to submit a report, no later than one year after the date of enactment, to Congress on the timeliness of payments by the VA to non-VA providers, among other things.[37]

Sec. 106. Reimbursement of Non-VA Providers Assigned to the Chief Business Office (CBO)

This section of the act requires the Secretary to transfer payment authority for hospital care, medical services, and other health care through non-VA providers, from the VISNs and VAMCs to the Chief Business Office (CBO) of VHA. This transfer will be effective on October 1, 2014. Furthermore, this section requires the VA, in each fiscal year that begins after the date of enactment, to include in VHA's CBO budget amounts to pay for hospital care, medical services, and other health care provided through non-VA providers and to exclude these amounts from the VISN and VAMC budgets.

---

[35] As amended by the Department of Veterans Affairs Expiring Authorities Act of 2014 (P.L. 113-175).

[36] 5 C.F.R. §1315. Also see, http://fms.treas.gov/prompt/regulations.html.

[37] As amended by the Department of Veterans Affairs Expiring Authorities Act of 2014 (P.L. 113-175).

TITLE II: HEALTH CARE ADMINISTRATIVE MATTERS

The major emphasis of this title is the requirement of several studies to examine a variety of issues pertaining to VA's health care delivery system, and to explore ideas on how best to reform the system.

Sec. 201. Independent Assessment of the VA Health Care Delivery Systems and Management Processes

This section requires the Secretary, no later than 90 days after enactment of the act, to contract with a private sector entity or entities to conduct an independent assessment of the hospital care, and medical services furnished in VA medical facilities. Among other things, the assessment must address current and projected demographics and unique health care needs of the patient population served by the VA; the VA's current and projected health care capabilities and resources; the appropriate system-wide access standard applicable to hospital care, medical services, and other health care furnished by and through the VA; the information technology strategies of the VA with respect to furnishing and managing health care; and the VA's processes for carrying out construction and maintenance projects at medical facilities and the medical facility leasing program. The Secretary is required to submit this assessment report to Congress and make it available to the public as well.

Sec. 202. Commission on Care

This section establishes a "Commission on Care" to undertake a comprehensive evaluation and assessment of veterans access to VA health care and strategically examine how best to organize the VHA. The "Commission on Care" will also examine how to locate health care resources and deliver health care to veterans during the 20-year period beginning on the date of the enactment of this act. The Commission will be composed of

15 voting members, and the appointment of Commissioners will be made not later than one year after the date of the enactment of this act by the Speaker of the House of Representatives, the Minority Leader of the House of Representatives, the Majority Leader of the Senate, the Minority Leader of the Senate, and the President of the United States. In appointing these Commissioners, at least one of the Commissioners must represent a Veteran Service Organization (VSO) recognized by the Secretary for the representation of veterans; have experience as senior manager for a private integrated health care system with an annual gross revenue of more than $50,000,000; be familiar with government health care systems, including those systems of the DOD, IHS, and FQHCs; be familiar with the VHA but not be a current employee of the VHA; and be familiar with medical facility construction and leasing projects carried out by government entities and have experience in the building trades, including construction, engineering, and architecture. The "Commission on Care" is required to submit to the President, through the Secretary, several reports on their findings. The final report should be submitted within 180 days of the initial commission meeting. This section requires the President to require the Secretary of Veterans Affairs and other heads of relevant executive departments and agencies to implement each recommendation included in the final report of the "Commission on Care," as specified.

Sec. 203. Technology Task Force on Review of Scheduling System and Software of the VA

This section requires the Secretary to conduct a review of the needs of the VA's scheduling system and scheduling software that is used to schedule appointments for veterans for hospital care, medical services, and other health care. The Secretary is required to use the free services of a technology task force for this purpose. Not later than 45 days after the date of the enactment of this act, the technology task force is required to submit to the Secretary and Congress a report setting forth the findings and recommendations of the technology task force regarding the needs of the

VA with respect to the scheduling system and scheduling software. Furthermore, this section requires the Secretary to make the report public no later than 30 days after the receipt of the report, and implement the recommendations in the report that the Secretary considers feasible, advisable, and cost effective.

Sec. 204. Improving Access to Mobile Vet Centers and Mobile Medical Centers

This section of the act requires the VA to provide standardized requirements to improve access of veterans to telemedicine services, other health care services, and readjustment counseling services provided by mobile Vet Centers and mobile medical centers. The standardized requirements include the number of days each mobile vet center and mobile medical center is expected to travel per year; the number of locations and events each center is expected to visit per year; the number of appointments and outreach contacts each center is expected to conduct per year; and the method and timing of notifications given by each center to individuals in the area to which the center is traveling, including notifications informing veterans of the availability to schedule appointments at the center. This section also requires the Secretary, one year after enactment, to submit an annual report (no later than September 30 of each year) to Congress outlining the recommended improvements for access to telemedicine, health care services, and readjustment counseling services through mobile Vet Centers and mobile medical centers, as well as data on the use of mobile Vet Centers and mobile medical centers.[38]

---

[38] As amended by the Department of Veterans Affairs Expiring Authorities Act of 2014 (P.L. 113-175).

Sec. 205. Improved Performance Metrics for Health Care Provided by the VA

This section of the act requires the Secretary to ensure that scheduling and wait-time metrics or goals are not used as factors in evaluating employee performance for purposes of determining whether to pay performance awards to the following categories of employees: directors, associate directors, assistant directors, deputy directors, chiefs of staff, and clinical leads of VA medical centers; and directors, assistant directors, and quality management officers of VISNs. Furthermore, no later than 30 days after enactment, the Secretary is required to modify the performance plans of the directors of the VA medical centers and the directors of the VISNs to ensure that performance plans are based on the quality of care received by the veterans, as specified. This section further stipulates that the Secretary must not include performance goals in the performance plans of VISN and medical center Directors that might provide incentives for not authorizing non-VA care furnished through non-VA entities.

Sec. 206. Improved Transparency Concerning Health Care Provided by the VA

This section requires the VA, no later than 90 days after the date of enactment, to publish in the *Federal Register*, and on a publicly accessible Internet website of each VA medical center, the wait-times for the scheduling of an appointment in that facility by a veteran for the receipt of primary care, specialty care, and hospital care and medical services based on the general severity of the condition of the veteran. Furthermore, whenever the wait-times for the scheduling of such an appointment changes, the Secretary is required to publish the revised wait-times on a publicly accessible Internet website of each VA medical center no later than 30 days after such a change; and in the *Federal Register* no later than 90 days after such change. This section also requires the Secretary to develop and make available to the public a comprehensive, machine-readable data set containing all applicable patient safety, quality of care, and outcome measures for health care provided by VA and tracked by the VA. Furthermore, at least once a year the VA is required to update the data. This section further stipulates that the Secretary must enter into an agreement with the Secretary of Health and Human Services (HHS) to provide VA hospital data on patient quality and outcomes as specified in order for it to be made available through the Hospital Compare Internet website of the Department of Health and Human Services (HHS). This section also requires the Government Accountability Office (GAO) to conduct a review, no later than three years after enactment of this act, of publicly available safety and quality metrics.[39]

Sec. 207. Information for Veterans on the Credentials of VA Physicians

This section requires the VA to improve the information available to veterans regarding residency training in the "Our Doctors" data set located on each VAMCs website. This section requires the VA to publish on its website the following information: name of the facility at which each VA physician underwent residency training, and identifying whether a physician is a physician in residency. Furthermore, this section stipulates that for those veterans undergoing surgical procedures, the VA is to provide them information on the education and training of the surgeon as well as the licensure, registration, and certification of the surgeon. This section of the act also requires the GAO to report to Congress on VA's Patient Centered Community Care program (PCCC) and requires the Secretary to submit a plan to Congress and to GAO in response to GAO's findings and recommendations, and to implement such recommendation no later than 90 days after submitting the report.[40]

---

[39] As amended by the Department of Veterans Affairs Expiring Authorities Act of 2014 (P.L. 113-175).

[40] As amended by the Department of Veterans Affairs Expiring Authorities Act of 2014 (P.L. 113-175).

Sec. 208. Information in Annual Budget of the President on Hospital Care and Medical Services Furnished through the Expanded Use of Contracts

This section requires that VA's annual congressional budget submissions include information pertaining to the number of veterans who received hospital care and medical services under the new expanded authority under Section 101 of P.L. 113-146; the amount expended by the VA on furnishing care and services under Section 101; the amount requested for the costs of furnishing care and services under Section 101; the number of veterans that the VA estimates will receive hospital care and medical services under Section 101 during the fiscal year of the budget request; and the number of VA employees on paid administrative leave at any point during the fiscal year preceding the fiscal year in which such budget request is submitted.

Sec. 209. Prohibition on Falsification of Data Concerning Wait Times and Quality Measures at the VA

This section of the act requires the Secretary to establish, no later than 60 days after enactment, policies that will impose penalties on VA employees who knowingly falsify data on patient wait-times or health care quality measures or knowingly request other VA employees to falsify such data.

TITLE III: HEALTH CARE STAFFING, RECRUITMENT, AND TRAINING MATTERS

The provisions of this title together aim to address the clinical workforce shortages in the VA health care system, and bolster recruitment and retention programs of the VA.

Sec. 301. Treatment of Staffing Shortage and Biennial Report on Staffing of VA Medical Facilities

This section requires the Inspector General (IG) to determine, and the Secretary to publish in the *Federal Register*, not later than September 30 annually, a list of the five VHA occupations, among the health professions listed in 38 U.S.C. §7401, that have the largest staffing shortages as calculated over the five year period that precedes the determination.[41] The section also specifies that the first determination be made and published not later than 180 days after enactment. The section also authorizes the Secretary to use the IG's determination to recruit and directly appoint qualified personnel in one of the identified occupations in the fiscal year that follows the report.

The section requires the Secretary to establish medical residency programs or to ensure that currently operating medical residency programs have sufficient positions at any VA facility that has a shortage or is located in a health professional shortage area as designated by the Department of Health and Human Services.[42] The subsection further requires that the Secretary allocate the residency positions among the occupations that the IG determined to be in shortage in the most recent report and must also give priority to residency positions in primary care, mental health, and any other specialty that the Secretary deems appropriate. The section also specifies that during the five-year period beginning on the day that is one year after enactment, the Secretary is required to increase the number of medical residency positions at VA facilities by up to 1,500 positions giving priority to medical facilities that do not, at the time of enactment, have a medical residency program and are located in a community that has a high concentration of veterans. Finally, the section requires that, on October 1 beginning in 2015 and continuing through 2019, the Secretary submit a report to the Committees on Veterans' Affairs in the House and Senate on VA graduate medical education that includes certain specified elements.

---

[41] The act adds a new §7412 to Subchapter 1 of Chapter 74 of title 38 U.S.C.
[42] The act adds a new §7302(e) to title 38 U.S.C. For more information about health professional shortage areas, see http://www.hrsa.gov/shortage/index.html.

The section amends the priority of the VA's *Scholarship Program of Health Professionals Educational Assistance Program to Certain Providers* to give priority to individuals who are in the final year of education or training in an occupation that the IG identified in its most recent determination as having a large staffing shortage.

The section also requires, not later than 180 days after enactment and not later than December 31 of each even-numbered year thereafter until 2024, that the Secretary submit to the Committees on Veterans' Affairs in the House and Senate a report that assesses staffing at each VHA facility. The report will also include assessments of the appropriateness of certain specified elements related to VA staffing, including but not limited to staffing levels, patient panel size,[43] workloads, and wait times in certain fields; staffing models used in these specified fields; succession planning at the VA, and the number of health providers who have left the VA during the two years that precede the report's submission, including the reason they have left the VA, among other things.[44]

Sec. 302. Extension and Modification of Certain Programs within the VA's Health Professionals Educational Assistance Program

This section extends authorization of the VA scholarship program until December 31, 2019. It also modifies the Education Debt Reduction program to increase the amount that the VA could pay in total to a participant, over a five-year period, from $60,000 to $120,000. It also increases the amount that could be paid in the fourth and fifth years from $12,000 to $24,000 per year. Finally, the section eliminates the requirement that VA education debt

---

[43] Generally the number of patients for a full-time physician provider.
[44] As amended by the Department of Veterans Affairs Expiring Authorities Act of 2014 (P.L. 113-175).

reduction payments may not exceed the amount of principal and interest that a participant owes during a single year.[45]

Sec. 303. Clinic Management Training for Employees at VA Medical Facilities

This section of the act requires the Secretary to commence a clinic management training program, no later than 180 days after the date of enactment of this act, to provide in-person, standardized education on systems and processes for health care practice management and scheduling to all appropriate employees at VA medical facilities. Among other things, the training must include how to manage the schedules of VA health care providers; training on the appropriate number of appointments that a health care provider should conduct on a daily basis, based on specialty; training on how to determine whether there are enough available appointment slots to manage demand for different appointment types and mechanisms for alerting management of insufficient slots; training on how to properly use the VA appointment scheduling system including any new scheduling system; training on how to optimize the use of technology; and training on how to properly use VA's physical plant space to ensure efficient flow and privacy for patients and staff. The training program must end on the date that is two years after the date on which the clinic management training program commences. After the termination of the program the Secretary is required to provide training materials and update them regularly.

TITLE IV: HEALTH CARE RELATED TO SEXUAL TRAUMA

This title liberalizes eligibility for VA sexual trauma counseling, care, and services to certain veterans and servicemembers.

---

[45] §408 of P.L. 113-175 further amends the Education Debt Reduction Program to permit the VA to directly make payments to the entities that hold the eligible individual's loans. As amended by the Department of Veterans Affairs Expiring Authorities Act of 2014 (P.L. 113-175).

Sec. 401. Expansion of Eligibility for Sexual Trauma Counseling and Treatment to Veterans on Inactive Duty Training

This section provides VA with the authority to provide counseling, care, and services to veterans, and certain other servicemembers who may not have veteran status, who experienced sexual trauma while serving on active duty for training or inactive duty for training.[46]

Sec. 402. Provision of Counseling and Treatment for Sexual Trauma by the VA to Members of the Armed Forces

This section amends Section 1720D of title 38, U.S.C., and allows the Secretary in consultation with the Secretary of Defense to provide counseling and treatment for sexual trauma victims in the Armed Forces (including members of the National Guard and Reserve components on active duty) without an initial consultation and referral from DOD.

Sec. 403. Reports on Military Sexual Trauma

This section requires the Secretary to submit various reports to Congress on Military Sexual Trauma.

TITLE V: OTHER HEALTH CARE MATTERS

This title extends the Assisted Living Pilot Program for Veterans with Traumatic Brain Injury until October 6, 2017.

---

[46] The act amends §1720D of title 38, U.S.C.

Sec. 501. Extension of Pilot Program on Assisted Living Services for Veterans with Traumatic Brain Injury

This section extends the pilot program established by Section 1705 of the National Defense Authorization Act (NDAA) for Fiscal Year 2008 (P.L. 110-181) through October 6, 2017. Section 1705 required the Secretary, in collaboration with DOD's Defense and Veterans Brain Injury Center (DVBIC), to carry out a five-year pilot program to assess the effectiveness of providing assisted living (AL) services to eligible veterans with traumatic brain injury (TBI). The AL-TBI pilot program was established for implementation between April 2008 and June 2013 and was administered through contracts with residential living programs designed to accommodate the needs of patients with TBI.

TITLE VI: MAJOR MEDICAL FACILITY LEASES

This title authorizes the VA to carry out specified major medical facility leases and requires the VA to comply with current laws and policies governing obligations for major medical facility leases.

Sec. 601. Authorization of Major Medical Facility Leases

This section of the act authorizes medical facility leases (requested by the VA in its FY2014 congressional budget submission) at the following locations: (1) Albuquerque, NM, for an amount of $9,560,000; (2) Brink, NJ, for an amount of $7,280,000; (3) Charleston, SC, for an amount of $7,070,250; (4) Cobb County, GA, for an amount of $6,409,000; (5) Honolulu, HI, for an amount of $15,887,370; (6) Johnson County, KS, for an amount of $2,263,000; (7) Lafayette, LA, for an amount of $2,996,000; (8) Lake Charles, LA, for an amount of $2,626,000; (9) New Port Richey, FL, for an amount of $11,927,000; (10) Ponce, PR, for an amount of $11,535,000; (11) San Antonio, TX, for an amount of $19,426,000; (12) San Diego, CA, for an amount of $11,946,100; (13) Tyler, TX, for an amount of $4,327,000; (14) West Haven, CT, for an amount of $4,883,000; (15) Worcester, MA, for an amount of $4,855,000; (16) Cape Girardeau, MO, for an amount of $4,232,060; (17) Chattanooga, TN, for an amount of $7,069,000; (18) Chico, CA, for an amount of $4,534,000; (19) Chula Vista, CA, for an amount of $3,714,000; (20) Hines, IL, for an amount of $22,032,000; (21) Houston, TX, for an amount of $6,142,000; (22) Lincoln, NE, for an amount of $7,178,400; (23) Lubbock, TX, for an amount of $8,554,000; (24) Myrtle Beach, SC, for an amount of $8,022,000; (25) Phoenix, AZ, for an amount of $20,757,000; (26) Redding, CA, for an amount of $8,154,000; and (27) Tulsa, OK, for an amount of $13,269,200.[47] This section also stipulates specific lease requirements for the leased clinic located in Tulsa, OK.[48]

Sec. 602. Budgetary Treatment of VA Major Medical Facilities Leases

This section requires the Secretary to record the full cost of the contractual obligation at the time a contract is executed either in an amount equal to total payments required under the full term of the lease; or equal to an amount sufficient to cover the first-year lease payments and any specified cancellation costs in the event that the lease is terminated before its full term. Furthermore, this section requires the VA to provide a detailed analysis of how such lease is expected to comply with Office of Management and Budget (OMB) Circular A–11 and Section 1341 of title 31, U.S.C. in a prospectus for a proposed lease, and requires the VA to submit to Congress the following information: (1) notice of the intent to enter into a lease; (2) a copy of the proposed lease; (3) an explanation of any difference between the prospectus and the lease submitted under this subsection; and (4) a scoring

---

[47] 38, U.S.C. §8104 requires that VA major medical facility leases, defined as "a lease for space for use as a new medical facility at an average annual rent of more than $1 million," be specifically authorized by law.

[48] These facilities are community based outpatient clinics (CBOCs). A VHA CBOC is a health care site that is geographically distinct and separate from a parent medical facility and may be a site that is VA-operated and/or contracted.

analysis demonstrating compliance with OMB Circular A–11. This information must be submitted to Congress not less than 30 days before entering into a major medical facility lease.

TITLE VII: OTHER VETERANS MATTERS

This section broadly address several areas including veterans education benefits, spending offsets, and provides authority for the removal or transfer of Senior Executive Service (SES) employees of the VA for performance or misconduct and requires expedited review of such actions.

Sec. 701. Expansion of Marine Gunnery Sergeant John David Fry Scholarship

This section expands eligibility for the Marine Gunnery Sergeant John David Fry Scholarship program to the spouse of an individual who, on or after September 11, 2001, dies in the line of duty while serving on active duty as a member of the Armed Forces.[49] Under this section a spouse would be entitled to the scholarship until the earlier of 15 years following the servicemember's death or remarriage. A similarly circumstanced spouse is currently eligible for educational assistance under the Survivors' and Dependents' Educational Assistance program (DEA). This section requires the spouse to make an irrevocable election to receive benefits under either the scholarship or DEA. The amendment is effective for terms beginning after December 31, 2014.[50]

---

[49] The Post-9/11 GI Bill provides educational assistance payments to eligible individuals enrolled in approved programs. Prior to the enactment of P.L. 113-146 the Marine Gunnery Sergeant John David Fry Scholarship program provided eligibility for the Post-9/11 GI Bill for the children of individuals who, on or after September 11, 2001, died in the line of duty while serving on active duty as a member of the Armed Forces.

[50] For more information on the Post-9/11 GI Bill, see CRS Report R42755, *The Post-9/11 Veterans Educational Assistance Act of 2008 (Post-9/11 GI Bill): Primer and Issues*, by Cassandria Dortch. For more information on DEA, see CRS Report R42785, *GI Bills Enacted Prior to*

Sec. 702. Approval of Courses of Education Provided by Public Institutions of Higher Learning for Purposes of All-Volunteer Force Educational Assistance Program and Post-9/11 Educational Assistance Conditional on In-State Tuition Rate for Veterans

This section requires the Secretary to disapprove a course at a public institution of higher learning (IHL) if the IHL charges tuition and fees above the in-state rate for that course to a qualifying Post-9/11 GI Bill or All-Volunteer Force Educational Assistance Program (MGIB-AD)[51] participant who is living in the state in which the IHL is located.[52] However, the public IHL may require the qualifying participant to demonstrate intent to establish residency, by a means other than physical presence, in order to qualify for in-state tuition. The course disapproval only applies to the Post-9/11 GI Bill and MGIB-AD. Qualifying Post-9/11 GI Bill and MGIB-AD participants are those who were discharged or released from a period of not fewer than 90 days of service in the *active military, naval, or air service* less than three years before the date of enrollment in said course and to their Post-9/11 GI Bill-eligible dependents and survivors.[53] If a course is disapproved, the qualifying participant cannot be approved for subsequent courses at the same IHL if continuously enrolled. This section is effective for terms beginning after July 1, 2015.[54]

2008 and Related Veterans' Educational Assistance Programs: A Primer, by Cassandria Dortch.

[51] The Post-9/11 GI Bill and MGIB-AD provide educational assistance payments to eligible individuals enrolled in approved programs. For more information on MGIB-AD, see CRS Report R42785, *GI Bills Enacted Prior to 2008 and Related Veterans' Educational Assistance Programs: A Primer*, by Cassandria Dortch.

[52] The Secretary may waive this requirement.

[53] The term "active military, naval, or air service," as defined in 38 U.S.C. §101(24), includes *active duty*. The term "active duty," as defined in 38 U.S.C. §101(21), is not equivalent to that defined in 38 U.S.C. §3301(1) or 38 U.S.C. §3002.

[54] As amended by the Department of Veterans Affairs Expiring Authorities Act of 2014 (P.L. 113-175).

Secs. 703, 704, 705, and 706

These sections of the act, respectively: extend the authorization period that requires the VA pension benefits for veterans and survivors who are residing in Medicaid-approved nursing homes to be reduced to $90 per month; extend the authorization period in which fees are charged from certain veterans for obtaining home-loan guarantees from the VA; limit the amount of awards or bonuses paid to VA employees; and extend the authorization period in which VA is required to obtain data from the Internal Revenue Service (IRS) and the Social Security Administration (SSA) to verify the income of VA pension applicants.

Sec. 707. Removal of Senior Executives of the VA for Performance or Misconduct

This section of the act provides the VA Secretary with new authority to remove senior executives from the department. The new authority and procedures created under this section apply to members of the Senior Executive Service (SES) in the VA, as well as individuals in certain leadership positions specific to the VA and commonly referred to as "Title 38 employees."[55] The new authority will be added to Title 38 of the U.S.C., which currently contains a set of adverse action procedures for employees appointed under that title, and is in addition to the authority the Secretary currently has to remove members of the SES under Title 5 of the U.S.C.[56]

---

[55] Title 38 U.S.C. employees covered by the act include "any individual who occupies an administrative or executive position and who was appointed under section 7306(a) or section 7401(1) of this title." Section 7306(a) of Title 38 establishes positions for administrative officials in the office of the under secretary for health, including several assistant undersecretaries for health, a director of physical assistant services, a director of nursing services, and several other administrative directors whose appointments are considered necessary to suit the needs of the department. Section 7401(1) includes "physicians, dentists, podiatrists, chiropractors, optometrists, registered nurses, physician assistants, and expanded-function dental auxiliaries."

[56] The act retains the Secretary's current authority for removing a member of the SES or a Title 38 employee. Under his current authority, the Secretary could instigate a removal for a member of the SES under 5 U.S.C. §3592, which allows him to remove a senior

If the Secretary determines that the performance of a senior executive warrants removal or that the individual has engaged in misconduct that warrants removal, he can invoke the authority provided in this section and remove a senior executive in one of two ways. First, the Secretary may remove the executive from the civil service entirely (i.e., from federal service). Second, the Secretary may transfer the executive into a position at any grade on the General Schedule (GS) "for which the individual is qualified and that the Secretary determines appropriate."[57] Under the second scenario, the individual would be compensated at the established rate for that position.[58]

If the Secretary chooses to remove an individual using this new authority, the Secretary must submit notice to the Senate and House Veterans' Affairs Committees within 30 days of the removal or transfer. The notice must contain the reasons for removal or transfer.

A removal or transfer made under this section would also be subject to a new set of expedited appeal procedures if the senior executive chose to appeal the Secretary's decision. First, the individual would have up to seven days to appeal the Secretary's decision to the Merit Systems Protection Board (MSPB). While the appeal is ongoing, the individual is not eligible for compensation, including pay, awards, bonuses, and other benefits.

Once the MSPB receives the appeal, the agency is to refer it to an administrative judge for review, and the judge has up to 21 days following the date of the appeal to issue a decision. To assist the MSPB in accomplishing the expedited review, the act instructs the Secretary to provide to the MSPB and the reviewing administrative judge "such information and assistance as may be necessary to ensure an appeal under

---

executive for unsatisfactory performance. In other circumstances, the Secretary could remove a member of the SES using adverse action procedures under 5 U.S.C. §7543 "for reasons of misconduct, neglect of duty, malfeasance, or failure to accept a directed reassignment or to accompany a position in a transfer of function." For individuals in the VA-specific positions created under Title 38, another set of adverse action procedures is available to the Secretary under that title (38 U.S.C. §§7461 *et seq.*).

[57] The General Schedule is the pay scale on which many white-collar employees in the civil service are compensated.

[58] Under current law, if an individual is removed from the SES for performance reasons, he or she is generally guaranteed placement into a GS-15 position and may be eligible to receive pay that is higher than what would otherwise have been allotted for that position. See 5 U.S.C. §3594(c)(1)(B).

this subsection is expedited." The administrative judge's decision is final and may not be subject to further appeal.

If the judge cannot issue a decision in the case within the required 21-day period, the Secretary's decision to remove or transfer the senior executive would become final. If such an instance were to occur, the MSPB must submit a report to the Senate and House Veterans' Affairs Committees explaining why the decision was not issued within 21 days.

This section also requires MSPB to establish a process to conduct these expedited reviews within 14 days of enactment of the act. The MSPB issued an interim final rule to comply with this requirement on August 19, 2014.[59] The rule is effective as of the date of issuance. Also within 14 days of enactment, the MSPB is required to report to the Committees on Veterans' Affairs in the Senate and House on their planned actions for expedited reviews. This report is to provide a description of the resources the MSPB expects will be necessary to conduct the reviews, including a description of any additional resources that may be necessary for the agency to fulfill its new responsibilities.

TITLE VIII: OTHER MATTERS

Sec. 801. Appropriation of Amounts

This section, among other things, authorizes and appropriates $5 billion for the VA to hire primary care and specialty care physicians and to hire other medical staff, including the following: physicians; nurses; social workers; mental health professionals; and other health care professionals as the Secretary considers appropriate. This funding will also be available for the maintenance and operation of VHA facilities including leases and minor construction.

---

[59] Merit Systems Protection Board, "Practices and Procedures; Appeal of Removal or Transfer of Senior Executive Service Employees of the Department of Veterans Affairs," 79 *Federal Register* 48941-48946, August 19, 2014; and Merit Systems Protection Board, "Practices and Procedures," 79 *Federal Register* 63031-63032, October 22, 2014.

Sec. 802. Veterans Choice Fund

This section establishes in the Treasury a new fund known as the "Veterans Choice Fund" and the Secretary will administer this fund. This section authorizes and appropriates $10 billion to be deposited in the Veterans Choice Fund, and this amount will be available until expended to implement only the provisions in Section 101. This section also stipulates that no more than $300 million of this amount shall be used for administrative expenses to implement Section 101.

The Surface Transportation and Veterans Health Care Choice Improvement Act of 2015 (H.R. 3236; P.L. 114-41) authorizes approximately $3.35 billion from the $10 billion deposited in the Veterans Choice Fund to be used for care outside the VA health care system, including $500 million of this amount for costs associated with prescription medications for the treatment of Hepatitis C.60 This authority expires on October 1, 2015.

Sec. 803. Emergency Designations

This section designates this act as an emergency requirement, and exempts it from budget enforcement rules.[61]

---

[60] Care outside the VA health care system (care provided in the community) includes care provided under the following statutory authorities (excluding the Veterans Choice Program): 38 U.S.C. §1703—non-VA medical care authority; 38 U.S.C. §1703note—Pilot Program Of Enhanced Contract Care Authority For Health Care Needs Of Veterans In Highly Rural Areas also known as Project ARCH (Access Received Closer to Home); 38 U.S.C. §1725—emergency care for nonservice-connected conditions; 38 U.S.C. §1728—emergency care for service-connected conditions; 38 U.S.C. §8111—sharing of health care resources with DOD and IHS; 38 U.S.C. §8153—contracts for health-care resources negotiated under this authority with institutions affiliated with VA under 38 U.S.C. §7302, including medical practice groups and other approved entities associated with affiliated institutions.

[61] Congress may exempt the budgetary effects of a provision in legislation from certain enforcement procedures by designating such provision as an emergency requirement. Under the existing budget enforcement rules, if a provision is so designated, the spending and revenue effects projected to result from that provision are not counted for purposes of enforcing the budget procedures. For more information see, CRS Report R41564, *Emergency Designation: Current Budget Rules and Procedures*, by Bill Heniff Jr.

APPENDIX. VETERANS ACCESS, CHOICE, AND ACCOUNTABILITY ACT OF 2014: IMPLEMENTATION AND REPORTING DEADLINES

Table A-1. Veterans Access, Choice, and Accountability Act of 2014 (P.L. 113-146 as Amended by P.L. 113-175 and P.L. 113-235): Implementation and Reporting Deadlines

Section of P.L. 113-146 as amended by P.L. 113-175 and P.L. 113-235	Brief Description	Implementation and/or Reporting Deadline[a]
Section 101(k)	The Secretary is required to implement an efficient nationwide system for processing and paying bills or claims for authorized care and services under the Veterans Choice Program. The Secretary is required to submit to the House and Senate Committees on Veterans' Affairs a quarterly report on the accuracy claims processing system.	The Secretary is required to prescribe regulations for the implementation of a claims processing system no later than November 5, 2014. Reports are due to the Committees no later than 20 days after the end of a quarter.
Section 101(n)	The Secretary is required to prescribe and publish interim final regulations on the implementation of Veterans Choice Program.	The Secretary is required to publish regulations in the *Federal Register* for the implementation of Veterans Choice Program no later than November 5, 2014.
Section 101(o)	The Inspector General of the VA is required to submit audit report to the Secretary.	The Inspector General's report is due no later than 30 days after the Secretary determines that 75% of the funds in the Veterans Choice Fund have been exhausted.

Section of P.L. 113-146 as amended by P.L. 113-175 and P.L. 113-235	Brief Description	Implementation and/or Reporting Deadline[a]
Section 101(p)	The authority to provide care and services under the Veterans Choice Program.	The authority for the Veterans Choice Program expires on August 7, 2017, or when funds in the Veterans Choice Fund have been exhausted—whichever occurs first.
		The Secretary is required to publish in the *Federal Register* and on the VA website a notice indicating expiration of the Veterans Choice Program. The Secretary is required to publish this notice 30 days before the funds are exhausted or no later than July 8, 2017.
Section 101(q)	The Secretary is required to submit to the House and Senate Committees on Veterans' Affairs a report on the furnishing of care and services under the Veterans Choice Program.	The initial report is due no later than February 3, 2015, and the final report is due no later than 30 days after the Secretary determines that 75% of the funds in the Veterans Choice Fund have been exhausted.
Section 101(s)	The Secretary is required to publish a report stating the actual wait-time goals of the VHA.	The Secretary is required to publish in the Federal Register and on a website a report stating the actual wait-time goals of the Veterans Health Administration no later than October 6, 2014.
Section 102(c)	The Secretary and the Director of the Indian Health Service are jointly required to submit a report to Congress regarding the enhancement of	The report is due to Congress no later than February 3, 2015.

Table A-1. (Continued)

Section of P.L. 113-146as amended by P.L. 113-175and P.L. 113-235	Brief Description	Implementation and/or Reporting Deadline[a]
	collaboration between the VA and Indian Health Service.	
Section 105(c)	The Government Accountability Office (GAO) is required to submit a report to Congress on the timeliness of payments by the VA for hospital care, medical services, and other health care furnished by non-VA health care providers.	The report is due to Congress no later than August 7, 2015.
Section 201(a)	The Secretary is required to enter into one or more contracts with a private sector entity or entities to conduct an independent assessment of the hospital care, medical services, and other health care furnished in VA medical facilities.	Contracts are required to be entered into no later than November 5, 2014. The assessment needs to be completed no later than July 3, 2015.
Section 201(d)	The program integrator is required to report the results of the independent assessment to the Secretary, the House and Senate Committees on Veterans' Affairs, and the Commission on Care.	The program integrator is required to report the results within 60 days of the assessment's conclusion. The Secretary is required to publish the results of the independent assessment in the Federal Registerand the VA website no later than 30 days after receiving the report.

Section of P.L. 113-146 as amended by P.L. 113-175 and P.L. 113-235	Brief Description	Implementation and/or Reporting Deadline[a]
Section 202(a)	Certain Members of the Congress holding leadership positions and the President are required to appoint a "Commission on Care" Majority of voting members of the "Commission on Care" appointed.	The Full Commission on Care needs to be established no later than August 7, 2015. A majority of the members of the Commission on Care must be appointed by February 18, 2015.
Section 202(b)	The Commission on Care is required to submit an interim and final report to the President, through the Secretary.	The Interim report is due no later than 90 days after the date of the initial meeting of the Commission on Care, and a final report not later than 180 days after the date of the initial meeting.
Section 202(g)	The President is required to submit a report to the House and Senate Committees on Veterans' Affairs and other appropriate committees on the recommendations contained in the Commission on Care report.	The report to the committees is due no later than 60 days after the President receives a report from the Commission on Care.
Section 203(a)	The Secretary is required to use a technology task force to conduct a review of the VA's patient scheduling system.	No specific deadline.
Section 203(b)	The technology task force is required to submit a report to the Secretary, the House and Senate Committees on Veterans' Affairs, regarding the needs of the VA with respect to the scheduling system and scheduling software.	The technology task force report is required no later than September 21, 2014. The Secretary is required to publish the technology task force report in the *Federal Register* and on the VA website no later than 30 days after receipt of the report.

Table A-1. (Continued)

Section of P.L. 113-146as amended by P.L. 113-175and P.L. 113-235	Brief Description	Implementation and/or Reporting Deadline[a]
Section 203(c)	The Secretary is required to implement the recommendations of technology task force report that the Secretary considers are feasible, advisable, and cost effective.	The Secretary is required to implement the recommendations nolater than one year after receipt of the report.
Section 204(b)	The Secretary is required to submit a report to the House and Senate Committees on Veterans' Affairs on access to care through VA mobile vet centers and mobile medical centers.	The Secretary is required to submit the report no later than August 7, 2015, and no later than September 30of eachyear thereafter.
Section 205(b)	The Secretary is required to modify the performance plans of the directors of the VAMCs and VISNs.	The Secretary is required to modify the performance plans no later than September 06, 2014.
Section 206(a)	The Secretary is required to publish the wait-times for the scheduling of an appointment at each VAMC for the receipt of primary care, specialty care, and hospital care and medical services based on the general severity of the condition of the veteran.	The Secretary is required to publish this information in the *Federal Register*and on a publicly accessible website no later than November 05, 2014. Whenever the wait-times for scheduling an appointment changes, the Secretary is required to publish the revised wait-times not later than 30 days after such change; and in the *Federal Register*by not later than 90 days after such change.
Section 206(b)	The Secretary is required to develop and make available to the public a comprehensive database containing patient safety, quality of care, and outcome measures for health care provided by the VA.	The Secretary is required to establish this database no later than February 3, 2015.

Section of P.L. 113-146 as amended by P.L. 113-175 and P.L. 113-235	Brief Description	Implementation and/or Reporting Deadline[a]
Section 206(c)	The Secretary is required to enter into an agreement with the Secretary of Health and Human Services for the provision of information to be available on the Hospital Compare Internet website.	The Secretary is required to enter into an agreement no later than February 3, 2015.
Section 206(d)	The Government Accountability Office (GAO) is required to conduct a review of the safety and quality metrics made publicly available by the VA.	The GAO is required to conduct the review no later than August 7, 2017.
Section 207(c)	The Government Accountability Office (GAO) is required to submit a report to the House and Senate Committees on Veterans' Affairs on the oversight of the credentialing of physicians under the Patient-Centered Community Care initiative as well the Veterans Choice Program.	The GAO report is required no later than August 7, 2016.
	The Secretary is required to submit a report to GAO and to the House and Senate Committees on Veterans' Affairs, a plan to address any findings and recommendations of the GAO report.	The plan is required no later than 30 days after the submittal of the GAO report.
		Secretary is required to implement the plan no later than 90 days after the submittal of the GAO report.
Section 209	The Secretary is required to establish policies that would impose penalties including termination of employees who knowingly submits false data concerning wait times for health care or quality	Secretary is required to implement these policies and penalties no later than October 6, 2014.

Table A-1. (Continued)

Section of P.L. 113-146as amended by P.L. 113-175and P.L. 113-235	Brief Description	Implementation and/or Reporting Deadline[a]
Section 301(a)	The VA Inspector General is required to determine, and the Secretary is required to publish the five medical occupations for which there are the largest staffing shortages throughout the VA.	The Secretary is required to publish in the Federal Registerthe VAInspector General's determination, no later than February 3, 2015, and by September 30 each year thereafter.
Section 301(b)	The Secretary is required to submit a report to the House and Senate Committees on Veterans' Affairs on graduate medical education residency positions at VA medical facilities.	The Secretary is required to submit this report on October 1 each year beginning 2015 and ending 2019.
Section 301(d)	The Secretary is required to submit a report to the House and Senate Committees on Veterans' Affairs assessing the staffing needs of each VA medical facility.	The Secretary is required to submit this report no later than February 3, 2015, and no later than December 31 of each even-numbered year thereafter until 2024.
Section 303(a)	The Secretary is required to implement a clinic management training program to provide in-person, standardized education on systems and processes for health care practice management and scheduling to all appropriate employees.	The Secretary is required to implement this clinic management training program no later than February 3, 2015.
Section 401	The act provides eligibility for sexual trauma counseling and treatment to veterans on inactive duty training.	Veterans on inactive duty training could receive services beginning August 7, 2014.

Section of P.L. 113-146 as amended by P.L. 113-175 and P.L. 113-235	Brief Description	Implementation and/or Reporting Deadline[a]
Section 402	The Secretary may, in consultation with the Secretary of Defense, provide sexual trauma counseling and treatment to members of the Armed Forces (including members of the National Guard and Reserves) on active duty.	Members of the Armed Forces (including members of the National Guard and Reserves) on active duty may receive services beginning August 7, 2015.
Section 403(a)	The Secretary is required to submit a report to the House and Senate Committees on Veterans' Affairs on VA services available for military sexual trauma.	The report on the treatment and services available from the VA for military sexual trauma is required to be submitted no later than April 28, 2016.
Section 403(b)	The Department of Veterans Affairs-Department of Defense Joint Executive Committee is required to submit a report to the House and Senate Committees on Veterans' Affairs on the transition of military sexual trauma treatment from DOD to VA.	The report on the transition of military sexual trauma treatment from DOD to VA must be submitted no later than April 28, 2016, and annually thereafter until September 30, 2021.
Section 501	Extension of Pilot Program on Assisted Living Services for Veterans with Traumatic Brain Injury.	The Assisted Living-Traumatic Brain Injury pilot will provided services to eligible veterans through contracts with private sector community-based and transitional rehabilitation programs from September 30, 2014, until October 6, 2017.
Section 601(b)	The Secretary is required to determine the most cost effective option over a 30-year life cycle for a CBOC in Tulsa, Oklahoma.	If the Secretary determines the most cost effective option is to construct a new CBOC the Secretary may request authority for a major medical facility project in Tulsa, Oklahoma, from Congress, and submit a detailed cost-benefit analysis no later than 90 days after making such a determination.

Table A-1. (Continued)

Section of P.L. 113-146as amended by P.L. 113-175and P.L. 113-235	Brief Description	Implementation and/or Reporting Deadline[a]
Section 602	The Secretary is required to submit reports to the House and Senate Committees on Veterans' Affairs on the budgetary treatment of VA major medical facilities leases.	The Secretary is required to submit a report no less than 30 daysbefore entering into a major medical facility lease and no more than 30 days after entering into a major medical facility lease.
Section 701	The act expands eligibility for the Marine Gunnery Sergeant John David Fry Scholarship program to the spouse of an individual who, on or after September 11, 2001, dies in the line of duty while serving on active duty as a member of the Armed Forces.	This is effective for terms beginning after December 31, 2014.
Section 702	The act requires the Secretary to disapprove a course at a public institution of higher learning (IHL) if the IHL charges tuition and fees above the in-state rate for that course to a qualifying Post-9/11 GI Bill or All-Volunteer Force Educational Assistance Program (MGIB-AD) participant who is living in the state in which the IHL is located.	This is effective for terms beginning after July 1, 2015.

Section of P.L. 113-146 as amended by P.L. 113-175 and P.L. 113-235	Brief Description	Implementation and/or Reporting Deadline[a]
Section 707	The act creates a new statute, 38 U.S.C. 713, which sets forth new rules for the removal or transfer of Senior Executive Service employees of the Department of Veterans Affairs (covered SES employees) for performance or misconduct and requires expedited review of such actions by the Merit Systems Protection Board.	The act requires the Merit Systems Protection Board to developand to put into effect expedited procedures for processing appeals filed pursuant to 38 U.S.C. 713 no later than August 21, 2014.
Section 801(d)	The Secretary is required submit a report to the House and Senate Veterans' Affairs Committees and Appropriations Committees, on how the VA has obligated the $5 billion that was authorized and appropriated to increase veterans access to care through the hiring of physicians and other medical staff and by improving VA's physical infrastructure.	The Secretary is required to submit the report no later than August 7, 2015.
Section 802(c)	The Secretary is required to submit a report to the House and Senate Veterans' Affairs and Appropriations Committees if the Secretary plans to use more than $300 million from the Veterans Choice Fund for administrative purposes to implement the Veterans Choice Program.	No specific deadline.

Source: Table prepared by the Congressional Research Service (CRS).

[a] Certain dates were calculated based on the number of days prescribed in P.L. 113-146 as amended by P.L. 113-175 and P.L. 113-235. Where the number of days is dependent upon certain preceding actions, only the number of days as indicated in the statute is presented. For example, if a report is due 90 days after an initial meeting, then only "90 days" is indicated.

In: The Veterans Choice Program (VCP)   ISBN: 978-1-53614-819-0
Editor: Mabel Page   © 2019 Nova Science Publishers, Inc.

Chapter 2

THE VETERANS CHOICE PROGRAM (VCP): PROGRAM IMPLEMENTATION*

Sidath Viranga Panangala

SUMMARY

Authorized under Section 101 of the Veterans Access, Choice, and Accountability Act of 2014 (VACAA), the Veterans Choice Program (VCP) is a new, temporary program that enables eligible veterans to receive medical care in the community. (P.L. 115-26 eliminated the August 7, 2017, expiration date for the VCP and allowed the program to continue until the initial $10 billion deposited in the Veterans Choice Fund was expended. The VA Choice and Quality Employment Act of 2017, P.L. 115-46, authorized and appropriated an additional $2.1 billion to continue the VCP until funds were expended, and when these funds were also nearing its end, Division D of P.L. 115-96 appropriated an additional $2.1 billion to continue the VCP until funds are expended.) It supplements several existing statutory authorities that allow the Veterans Health Administration (VHA) to provide health care services to veterans outside of the Department of Veterans Affairs (VA) facilities. Generally, all medical care

---

* This is an edited, reformatted and augmented version of Congressional Research Service, Publication No. R44562, dated April 20, 2018.

and services (including inpatient, outpatient, pharmacy, and ancillary services) are provided through the VCP—institutional long-term care and emergency care in non-VA facilities are excluded from the VCP and are provided under different authorities. The VCP is not a health insurance plan for veterans, nor does it guarantee health care coverage to all veterans.

Eligibility and Choice of Care. Veterans must be enrolled in the VA health care system to request health services under the VCP. A veteran may request a VA community care consult/referral, or his or her VA provider may submit a VA community care consult/referral to the VA Care Coordination staff within the VA.

Veterans may become eligible for the VCP in one of four ways. First, a veteran is informed by a local VA medical facility that an appointment cannot be scheduled within 30 days of the clinically determined date requested by his or her VA doctor *or* within 30 days of the date requested by the veteran (this category also includes care not offered at a veterans' primary VA facility and a referral cannot be made to another VA medical facility or other federal facility). Second, the veteran lives 40 miles or more from a VA medical facility that has a full-time primary care physician. Third, the veteran lives 40 miles or less (not residing in Guam, America Samoa, or the Republic of the Philippines) *and* either travels by air, boat, or ferry to seek care from his or her local facility *or* incurs a traveling burden of a medical condition, geographic challenge, or an environmental factor. Fourth, the veteran resides 20 miles or more from a VA medical facility located in Alaska, Hawaii, New Hampshire (excluding those who live 20 miles from the White River Junction VAMC), or a U.S. territory, with the exception of Puerto Rico.

Once found eligible for care through the VCP, veterans may choose to receive care from a VA provider *or* from an eligible VA community care provider (VCP provider). VCP providers are federally-qualified health centers, Department of Defense (DOD) facilities, or Indian Health Service facilities, and hospitals, physicians, and nonphysician practitioners or entities participating in the Medicare or Medicaid program, among others. A veteran has the choice to switch between a VA provider and VCP provider at any time.

Program Administration and Provider Participation. The VCP is administered by two third-party administrators (TPAs): Health Net and TriWest. Generally, Health Net and TriWest manage veterans' appointments, counseling services, card distributions, and a call center. The TPAs contract directly with the VA. Then, Health Net or TriWest will contract with eligible non-VA community care providers interested on participating in the VCP. At the end of September 2018, the VA has announced that it would end its contract with Health Net as a TPA because of low patient volume, customer service issues and late payments to community providers in its network. It is anticipated that TriWest would continue to be a TPA for the areas they manage.

Payments. Generally, a veteran's out-of-pocket costs under the VCP are equal to VHA out-of-pocket costs. Veterans do not pay any copayments at the time of their medical appointments. Copayment rates are determined by the VA after services are furnished. Enactment of P.L. 115-26 on April 19, 2017, allowed VA to become the primary payer when certain veterans with other health insurance (OHI) receive care for nonservice-connected conditions under VCP—veterans would not have to pay a copayment under their OHI anymore. The VA would coordinate with a veteran's OHI and bill for any copayments that the veteran would be responsible for similar to what they would have paid had they received care within a VA medical facility. Participating community providers are reimbursed by their respective TPA, and VA pays the TPAs.

INTRODUCTION

In response to concerns about access to medical care at many Department of Veterans Affairs (VA) hospitals and clinics across the country in spring 2014,[1] Congress passed the Veterans Access, Choice, and Accountability Act of 2014 (VACAA, P.L. 113-146, as amended). On August 7, 2014, President Obama signed the bill into law.[2] Since the VCAA was enacted, Congress has amended the act several times: P.L. 113-175, P.L. 113-235, P.L. 114-9, P.L. 114-41, P.L. 115-26, P.L. 115-46, and P.L. 115-96. In addition, the VA has issued implementation regulations and guidance on several occasions in response to the changes to VACAA and challenges encountered during implantation of the law. *Table 1* provides major highlights pertaining to the Veterans Choice Program (VCP)—a new,

---

[1] Department of Veterans Affairs, Office of Inspector General, *Review of Alleged Patient Deaths, Patient Wait Times, and Scheduling Practices at the Phoenix VA Health Care System*, 14-02603-267, August 26, 2014. For a summary of wait-time issues at a VA medical facility, by state, see Department of Veterans Affairs Office of Inspector General, *Administrative Summaries of Investigation Regarding Wait Times*, http://www.va.gov/oig/publications/administrativesummaries-of-investigation.asp Accessed on November 14, 2017.

[2] P.L. 113-146 as amended by P.L. 113-175, P.L. 113-235, P.L. 114-9, and P.L. 114-41. For a detailed provision-byprovision explanation of the act, see CRS Report R43704, *Veterans Access, Choice, and Accountability Act of 2014 (H.R. 3230; P.L. 113-146)*.

temporary program that allows eligible veterans to receive medical care in the community authorized by Section 101 of the VACAA.

Table 1. Veterans Choice Program (VCP) Timeline

Date	Action
August 7, 2014	The Veterans Access, Choice, and Accountability Act of 2014 (P.L. 113-146) signed into law. The Secretary is required to publish regulations in the Federal Register for the implementation of Veterans Choice Program (VCP) no later than November 5, 2014.
September 26, 2014	The Department of Veterans Affairs Expiring Authorities Act of 2014 (P.L. 113-175) was signed into law. The act makes several technical amendments to the Veterans Access, Choice, and Accountability Act of 2014 (P.L. 113-146).
November 5, 2014	The Department of Veterans Affairs issues interim final rules implementing the Veterans Choice Program (VCP). VA begins mailing out a Choice Card to every enrolled veteran and every separating servicemember.
December 16, 2014	The Consolidated and Further Continuing Appropriations Act, 2015 (P.L. 113-235) is signed into law. The act made several technical amendments allowing the VA to reimburse providers in the state of Alaska, under the VA Alaska Fee Schedule, and in states with an "All-Payer Model" agreement, VA was allowed to calculate Medicare payments based on payment rates under such "All-Payer Model" agreements.
April 24, 2015	The Department of Veterans Affairs issues interim final rules modifying how VA measures the distance from a veteran's residence to the nearest VA medical facility. This modification considered the distance the veteran must drive to the nearest VA medical facility from the veterans' residence, rather than the straightline or geodesic distance to VA facility.
May 12, 2015	Department of Veterans Affairs issues memorandum to Veterans Integrated Service Network (VISN) Directors on VA Care in the Community (Non-VA Purchased Care) and use of the Veterans Choice Program. The memorandum outlines that effective June 8, 2015, a specific hierarchy of care must be used when the veteran's primary VA medical facility cannot readily provide needed care to a veteran, either because the

Date	Action
	care is unavailable at the facility or because the facility cannot meet VHA's wait time criteria.
May 22, 2015	The Construction Authorization and Choice Improvement Act was signed into law (P.L. 114-19) and amended the 40 miles eligibility criteria for the Veterans Choice Program (VCP) to clarify that the 40 miles is calculated based on distance traveled (driving distance) rather than the previous straight-line or geodesic distance standard, and authorized VA to determine if there is an unusual or excessive burden in traveling to a VA medical facility.
July 31, 2015	The Surface Transportation and Veterans Health Care Choice Improvement Act (P.L. 114-41) is signed into law. Among other things the act allowed all enrolled veterans to be eligible for the Veterans Choice Program (amended the August 1, 2014 enrollment date restriction), defined the nearest VA medical facility as a Community Based Outpatient Clinic (CBOC) with no full time primary care physician, removed the 60-day limitation on an episode of care, included clinically indicated date as a wait time eligibility criteria, and expanded provider eligibility.
October 1, 2015	Department of Veterans Affairs issues memorandum to Veterans Integrated Service Network (VISN) Directors on VA Care in the Community (Non-VA Purchased Care) and use of the Veterans Choice Program that modifies the May 12, 2015 memorandum. The memorandum provides guidance on the hierarchy of care in the Veterans Choice Program (VCP). This allows VA medical facilities to refer the veteran to VCP for care not available at the veterans' primary VA medical facility and for which a referral pattern does not exist to another VA medical facility or other federal facility.
October 29, 2015	The Department of Veterans Affairs (VA) publishes final rules based on interim final rules published on November 5, 2014 and on April 24, 2015. These rules don't incorporate amendments to the Veterans Choice Program (VCP) made by the Surface Transportation and Veterans Health Care Choice Improvement Act (P.L. 114-41).
December 1, 2015	The Department of Veterans Affairs (VA) publishes interim final rules revising previous VA regulations implementing the Veterans Choice Program (VCP) based on amendments made by The Construction Authorization and Choice Improvement

Table 1. (Continued)

Date	Action
December 1, 2015	Act was signed into law (P.L. 114-19) and the Surface Transportation and Veterans Health Care Choice Improvement Act (P.L. 114-41).
April 19, 2017	P.L. 115-26 (unofficially referred to as the Veterans Choice Program Improvement Act), eliminates the August 7, 2017, sunset date of the Veterans Choice Program (VCP) and authorizes the program to continue until all the funds in the Veterans Choice Fund established by Section 802 of the Veterans Access, Choice, and Accountability Act of 2014 are expended. Furthermore, P.L. 115-26 authorized the Department of Veterans Affairs (VA) to become the primary payer for veterans with other health insurance (OHI) for care or services related to a nonservice-connected disability for which the veteran is entitled to care under the veteran's OHI. The VA would coordinate with the veteran's OHI and bill for any copayments that the veteran would be responsible for similar to what they would have paid had they received medical care or services within a VA medical facility.
August 12, 2017	The VA Choice and Quality Employment Act of 2017 (P.L. 115-46) authorized and appropriated $2.1 billion for the Veterans Choice Fund (established by Section 802 of the Veterans Access, Choice, and Accountability Act of 2014). Funds would remain available until expended.
December 20, 2017	The VA publishes a notice in the *Federal Register* indicating that all amounts deposited in the Veterans Choice Fund would be exhausted sometime between January 2, 2018, and January 16, 2018.
December 22, 2017	The President signed into law P.L. 115-96 (an Act to amend the Homeland Security Act of 2002 to require the Secretary of Homeland Security to issue Department of Homeland Security-wide guidance and develop training programs as part of the Department of Homeland Security Blue Campaign, and for other purposes). Division D of P.L. 115-96 appropriated an additional $2.1 billion for the Veterans Choice Fund. Funds would remain available until expended.

The VCP supplements several already existing statutory authorities[3] that allow the VA to provide care outside of its own health care system. These existing statutory authorities are briefly described in *Table A-1*. Congress has continued to keep the VCP funded and authorized, and has indicated that it plans to continue the program, until a streamlined and permanent care in the community program is authorized to replace this temporary program.[4] The Senate and House Veterans Affairs Committees have reported two measures to amend current law and to establish a new permanent care in the community program. On December 5, 2017, the Senate Veterans Affairs Committee reported the "Caring for our Veterans Act of 2017" (S. 2193; S.Rept. 115- 212),[5] and on March 5, 2018, "VA Care in the Community Act" (H.R. 4242; H.Rept. 115-585) was reported with an amendment by the House Veterans' Affairs Committee.[6]

This report provides details on how the VCP is being implemented. It is meant to provide insight into the execution of the current VCP program.

Scope and Limitations

Information contained in this chapter is drawn from regulations published in the *Federal Register*, conference calls and numerous meetings with VHA staff, and briefing materials and other information provided by the VA Office of Government Relations (which may not be publicly available). This chapter does not discuss the numerous issues that have

---

[3] For a complete summary of the VA Care in the Community programs, see, CRS Report R42747, *Health Care for Veterans: Answers to Frequently Asked Questions*.

[4] "Department of Homeland Security Blue Campaign Authorization Act of 2017," Remarks by Representative David P. Roe, *Congressional Record*, vol. 163 (December 21, 2017), p. H10399.

[5] On November 29, 2017, the Senate Committee on Veterans' Affairs marked up a draft measure, and it was reported to the Senate on December 5, 2017(without a written report), titled Caring for our Veterans Act of 2017 (S. 2193). Subsequently a written report (S.Rept. 115-212) was filed on March 7, 2018.

[6] On November 3, 2017, the VA Care in the Community Act, 2017 (H.R. 4242) was introduced, and the measure was marked up and ordered to be reported as amended on December 19, 2017. The bill was reported from the committee on March 5, 2018.

arisen during the implementation of VCP or legislative proposals currently under consideration in Congress to replace the VCP.

MEDICAL SERVICES UNDER VCP

Once an eligible veteran is authorized to receive necessary treatment, including follow-up appointments and ancillary and specialty medical services, under the VCP, a veteran may receive similar services that are offered through their personalized standard medical benefits package at a VA facility. VA's standard medical benefits package includes (but is not limited to) inpatient and outpatient medical, surgical, and mental health care; pharmaceuticals; pregnancy and delivery services; dental care; and durable medical equipment, and prosthetic devices, among other things.[7] Currently, 81 categories of medical services and procedures are authorized to be provided under VCP.[8] However, institutional long-term care and emergency

---

[7] For a complete summary of the VA's standard medical benefits package, see CRS Report R42747, *Health Care for Veterans: Answers to Frequently Asked Questions*; and 38 C.F.R. §17.38.

[8] The 81 categories of medical services and procedures covered in the community under the VCP are acupuncture; allergy and immunology; audiology; biofeedback; cardiology catheterization; cardiology imaging; cardiology rehabilitation; cardiology stress test; cardiology tests, procedures, studies; chemotherapy; chiropractic; colonoscopy; dental; dermatology; dermatology tests, procedures, studies; endocrinology; endocrinology tests, procedures, studies; ear, nose, and throat; gastroenterology; gastroenterology tests, procedures, studies; genetic testing/counseling; gynecology; gynecology tests, procedures, studies; hematology/oncology; Hepatitis C; homemaker home health aid; hospice; hyperbaric therapy; infectious disease; interventional radiology; intravenous therapy (IV)/ infusion, clinic; lab and pathology; medicine; mental health; nephrology; neurology; neurology tests, procedures, studies; neuropsych testing; neurosurgery; newborn care; noninstitutional IV/infusion care; noninstitutional skilled home care; noninstitutional skilled nursing care; noninstitutional spinal cord care; nuclear medicine; nutrition/dietitian services; obstetrics; occupational therapy; ophthalmology; ophthalmology tests, procedures, studies; optometry; orthopedic; orthopedic tests, procedures, studies; pain management; physical therapy; plastic surgery; podiatry; primary care; pulmonary; pulmonary rehabilitation; pulmonary tests, procedures, studies; radiation therapy; radiology; radiology CT scan; radiology DEXA scan; radiology mammogram; radiology MRI/MRA; radiology PET scan; radiology ultrasound; rehabilitation medicine; respiratory therapy; rheumatology; sleep study/polysomnography; surgery general; thoracic surgery; urology; urology tests, procedures, studies; vascular; vascular tests, procedures, studies; veteran directed home and community based services; and wound care (Source: Department of Veterans Affairs, FY2018 Congressional Budget Submission, *Medical Programs and Information Technology Programs,* vol. 2 of 4, May 2017, pp. VHA-319- VHA- 320).

care in non-VA facilities are excluded from the VCP. "It is important to note that the VCP does not provide guaranteed health care coverage or an unlimited medical benefit."[9] These services are authorized and provided under separate statutory authorities outside the scope of VCP (see *Table A-1*).

ELIGIBILITY

Generally, all veterans have to be enrolled in the VA health care system[10] to receive care under the VCP. Once this initial criterion is met, a qualified veteran may choose to receive care through VCP. Veterans may become eligible for care under the VCP through one of four different pathways[11]

- 30-day wait list (Wait-Time Eligible): A veteran is eligible for care through the VCP when he or she is informed, by a local VA medical facility, that an appointment cannot be scheduled
  - within 30 days of the clinically determined date of when the veteran's provider determines that he or she needs to be seen (this category also includes care not offered at the veterans' primary VA medical facility and a referral cannot be made to another VA medical facility or federal facility),[12] *or*
  - within 30 days of the date of when the veteran wishes to be seen.

---

[9] Letter from Veterans Health Administration, Chief Business Office Purchased Care to Veteran, Eligible Choice 30- Day Wait Recipient, September 25, 2015.

[10] For general enrollment procedures, see CRS Report R42747, *Health Care for Veterans: Answers to Frequently Asked Questions*.

[11] Department of Veterans Affairs, "Expanded Access to Non-VA Care through the Veterans Choice Program," 80 *Federal Register* 74991-74996, December 1, 2015 (codified at 38 C.F.R.§17.1510).

[12] Department of Veterans Affairs, *VA Care in the Community (Non-VA Purchased Care) and use of the Veterans Choice Program*, Memorandum from Acting Principal Deputy Under Secretary for Health to Veterans Integrated Service Network (VISN) Directors, May 12, 2015, and amended on October 1, 2015.

- 40 miles or more distance (Mileage Eligible): A veteran is eligible for care through the VCP when he or she lives 40 miles or more from a VA medical facility that has a full-time primary care physician.
- 40 miles or less distance (Mileage Eligible): A veteran is eligible for care through the VCP when he or she resides in a location, other than one in Guam, American Samoa, or the Republic of the Philippines, and
  o travels by air, boat, or ferry in order to seek care from his or her local VA facility; or
  o incurs a traveling burden[13] based on environmental factors, geographic challenges, or a medical condition.[14]
- State or territory without a full-service VA medical facility: A veteran is eligible for care through the VCP when his or her residence is more than 20 miles from a VA medical facility and located in either
  o Alaska,
  o Hawaii,
  o New Hampshire (excluding veterans who live 20 miles from the White River Junction VAMC), or
  o U.S. territory (excluding Puerto Rico).

A veteran who believes that he or she meets one of the eligibility criteria to receive care through the VCP is to have his or her eligibility status confirmed by local VA staff. A high level overview of the eligibility process to access care through the VCP is illustrated in *Figure 1*. Local VA facility

---

[13] Local VA staff decides whether or not the burden is unusual or excessive and likely to exist "at least 30 days or more from the date of the determination." Staff are to document the decision on VA Form 119, Report of Contact, which includes the date of determination, expected duration of travel burden, and reason(s) behind the decision. Notification is to be sent in a letter by mail to the veteran. Department of Veterans Affairs, Veterans Health Administration, *Veterans Choice Program - Unusual or Excessive Burden Determination*, September 11, 2015.

[14] A local VA provider or the facility's Primary Care Patient Aligned Care Team (PACT) determines whether or not a veteran is facing an unusual or excessive travel burden due to a medical condition. The duration of the burden is also assessed.

staff members are to review clinical and administrative records of the veteran to determine the appropriate medical benefits package and clinical criterion. Confirmation of the veteran's eligibility status is generally determined within 10 business days from when the request for confirmation was submitted. Veterans who are found ineligible to participate in the VCP are to be given instructions, in their notification letters, on how to appeal the VA's decision.[15]

CHOICE OF CARE

Eligible veterans have two options for receiving health care services under the Veterans Choice Program (VCP). First, veterans may choose to receive their medical care from a VA provider. A veteran who chooses this option is to receive an appointment with a VA provider. The veteran may be offered a VA appointment that is more than 30 days out or at a facility that is more than 40 miles from the veteran's residence.[16] If an offered appointment does not accommodate the veteran's clinical needs, the local VA staff may place the veteran on an electronic waiting list until an alternate appointment becomes available. *At any time*, the veteran (based on the availability of clinical appointments) may choose to receive his or her medical services from a VA community care provider.

The second option allows veterans to receive health care services from a VA community care provider (VCP provider) who accepts eligible VCP veterans. Veterans who choose this option are to have their names and medical authorization information sent to a VCP provider of their choice.[17]

---

[15] Veterans may appeal the decision of their local facility to the Board of Veterans Appeals (BVA). First, veterans would send a notice of disagreement to their facility. Then the facility is to generate a statement of case (SOC). Lastly, the facility is to process the appeal and forward it to the BVA for processing. Department of Veterans Affairs, Veterans Health Administration, *Veterans Choice Program - Unusual or Excessive Burden Determination*, September 11, 2015, p. 3.

[16] Department of Veterans Affairs, "Expanded Access to Non-VA through the Veterans Choice Program," 79 *Federal Register* 65577, November 5, 2014 (codified at 38 C.F.R. §17.1515).

[17] 38 C.F.R. §17.1515.

At any time, veterans (based on the availability of clinical appointments) may choose to receive their medical services from a VA provider.

> **Two Options to Choosing Care under the Veterans Choice Program (VCP)**
>
> Based on the availability of appointments,
> - A veteran may choose to receive medical care from a VA provider.
> - A veteran may choose to receive medical care from a VA community care provider.

VCP PROVIDERS

Under the VCP several entities and providers are eligible to provide care and services. These include among others, federally-qualified health centers, Department of Defense (DOD) medical facilities, Indian Health Service outpatient health facilities or facilities operated by a tribe or tribal organization, hospitals, physicians, and nonphysician practitioners or entities participating in the Medicare or Medicaid program, an Aging and Disability Resource Center, an area agency on aging, or a state agency or a center for independent living. VA employees are excluded from providing care or services under VCP, unless the provider is an employee of VA, and is not acting within the scope of such employment while providing hospital care or medical services through the VCP.[18] Generally, VCP providers "must maintain at least the same or similar credentials and licenses as those required of VA's health care providers."[19]

---

[18] 38 C.F.R. §17.1530.
[19] 38 C.F.R. §17.1530.

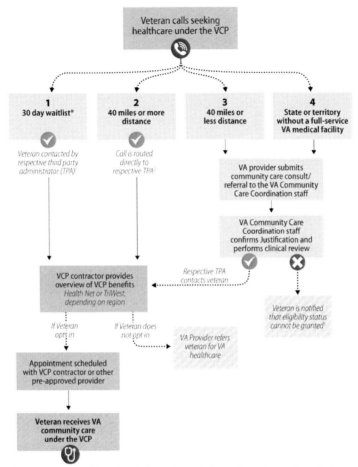

Source: Figure prepared by CRS based on information from the Veterans Health Administration.

Notes: * this category includes care not offered at the veterans' primary VA medical facility and a referral cannot be made to another VA medical facility or federal facility. Illustrated is a high level overview of the process to access care under the Veterans Choice Program (VCP). This figure does not specify (1) the criteria VA staff uses to determine veterans' eligibility statuses; (2) the interactions veterans will encounter throughout their processes to access care under the VCP; or (3) how local VA Medical Centers (VAMC) may enter into provider agreements with VA community care providers. This figure does not reflect the appeals process.

Figure 1. Eligibility Process to Access Care through the Veterans Choice Program (VCP).

PROGRAM ADMINISTRATION

The Veterans Choice Program (VCP) is not a health insurance plan for veterans. Under the VCP, veterans are given the option of receiving care in their local communities instead of waiting for a VA appointment and/or enduring traveling burdens to reach a VA facility.[20]

All veterans who are enrolled in the VA health care system are to be mailed a VCP card. The card lists relevant information about the VCP. Many veterans have attempted to use the VCP card as an insurance card. The VCP card may not be used to pay for medical services performed outside of or within the VA. Specifically, the VCP card does not

- replace veterans' identification cards,
- guarantee eligibility under the VCP,[21] or
- provide health insurance-like benefits (i.e., the VCP, like all VA health care, is not health insurance).

Third-Party Administrators (TPAs)

In September 2013, the VA awarded contracts to Health Net[22] and TriWest[23] to expand veterans' access to non-VA health care in the community, under the Patient-Centered Community Care (PC3) initiative.[24]

---

[20] Secretary Robert A. McDonald, *An Open Letter to America's Veterans*, Department of Veterans Affairs, Veterans Health Administration, 2014, http://www.va.gov/opa/choiceact/documents/Open-Letter-to-Veterans.pdf. Accessed on December 29, 2017.

[21] Department of Veterans Affairs, *Veterans Choice Program, Leadership Toolkit for VA Facilities*, p. 16.

[22] Health Net Federal Services, *Overview of Health Net Federal Services' VA Programs*, https://www.hnfs.com/   content/hnfs/home/company/company-information/va.html. Accessed on December 29, 2017.

[23] TriWest Healthcare Alliance, http://www.triwest.com/en/veteran-services/veterans-choice-program-vcp/. Accessed on January 2, 2018.

[24] The Patient-Centered Community Care (PC3) initiative evolved from the Project on Healthcare Effectiveness through Resource Optimization (Project HERO) pilot program. Under the PC3 program, VA provides contracted inpatient and outpatient specialty care and mental health care to eligible veterans when VA medical facilities

Later, in November 2014, the VA modified those contracts to include support services under the Veterans Access, Choice, and Accountability Act of 2014 (VACAA, or the Choice Act). Under the Veterans Choice Program (VCP), Health Net and TriWest manage the appointments, counseling services, card distributions, and a call center.[25] They also oversee VCP providers, medical services reporting and billing processes, and the coordination of care with private health insurers. As illustrated in *Figure 2*, Health Net covers Regions 1, 2, and 4, and TriWest covers Regions 3, 5A, 5B, and 6. In March 2018, the VA announced that the VCP contract with Health Net would end by September 2018 (see text box below). Low volume of patients, customer service issues and delayed payments to community providers were potentially some of the reasons for this decision.[26]

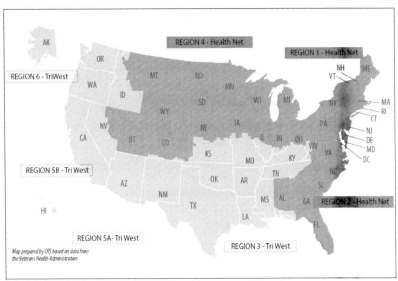

Source: Map prepared by CRS based on data from the Veterans Health Administration.

Figure 2. VCP Regions Covered by Third-Party Administrators.

---

cannot provide services such as when there is a lack of medical specialists, or long wait times, or there is an extraordinary long distance from the veteran's residence.

[25] Veterans Health Administration, *Choice Champion Call*, November 10, 2015, p. 31.

[26] Senate Committee on Veterans' Affairs, "Tester, Crapo Hold Health Net Accountable For 'Poor Performance," press release, March 13, 2013, https://www.veterans.senate.gov/newsroom/minority-news/tester-crapo-hold-health-netaccountable-for-poor-performance, and https://www.veterans.senate.gov/download/shulkin-re-health-net. Accessed April 18, 2018.

Contract with Health Net Federal Services

The VA plans not to renew the contract with Health Net as the TPA for the VCP after its scheduled end date of September 30, 2018. The Department stated that it has been increasingly utilizing provider agreements (Department Of Veterans Affairs Veterans Health Administration (VHA) Veterans Choice Program Provider Agreement; VA Form 10-10145) directly with community providers under the VCP, and therefore no longer needs the services of Health Net (those community providers who wish to be a VCP provider would have the option of establishing provider agreement directly with the VA). According to the VA, after the contract with Health Net ends, the VA would be directly responsible for the authorization of care, coordination of appointments, and payments to community providers. Currently scheduled medical appointments through the Health Net community network would take place until September 30, 2018. Appointments scheduled after this date would be transitioned back to VA and would be rescheduled with community providers using provider agreements. The TPA contract with TriWest would not be affected at this time.

Source: Department of Veterans Affairs, "Contract with Health Net Federal Services to End," Fact Sheet, March 2018.

Community Care Provider Participation[27]

Eligible non-VA community care providers may become VCP providers. Providers who are interested in participating in the VCP may do so either through the Patient Centered Community Care (PC3) network or the Choice network. Community providers who are under the Choice

---

[27] Major portions of this section are adapted from, Department of Veterans Affairs, Veterans Health Administration, How to become a Veterans Choice Program and/or Patient-Centered Community Care Provider, VA Community Care Fact Sheet for Interested Providers, May 24, 2017, p. 2. https://www.va.gov/opa/choiceact/documents/How_to_Become_VA_ Provider_05242017_508.pdf. Details on how providers could participate in VCP are available at https://www.va.gov/opa/choiceact/for_providers.asp. Accessed on January 2, 2018.

network may only render authorized services to VCP-eligible veterans. Under the PC3 network, all veterans who are eligible for VA community care may be seen.[28] The reason is that there are two different statutory authorities for care delivered through VCP and PC3. Interested providers are required to contact Health Net and/or TriWest to determine whether they qualify as a VA community care provider.[29] To qualify, providers must meet the following criteria:

- Have a full, current, and unrestricted state license and the same/similar VA credentials.
- Not be named on the Centers for Medicare and Medicaid Services (CMS) exclusionary list.[30]
- Meet all Medicare Conditions of Participation (CoPs) and Conditions for Coverage (CfCs).[31]
- Accept Medicare or Medicaid rates.
- Provide resources (services, facilities, and providers) that are in compliance with applicable federal and state regulatory requirements.
- Submit all medical records of rendered services to veterans to the TPA for inclusion in veterans' VA electronic medical records.

---

[28] Under the PC3 program, VA provides contracted inpatient and outpatient specialty care and mental health care to eligible veterans when VA medical facilities cannot provide services such as when there is a lack of medical specialists, or long wait times, or there is an extraordinary long distance from the veteran's residence.

[29] Health Net may be contacted by phone (1-866-606-8198; press Option 2) or email (HNFSProviderRelations@Healthnet.com). Accessed on January 2, 2018. TriWest may be contacted by phone (1-866 284-3743) or email (TriWestDirectContracting@triwest.com). For additional information about TriWest, see https://www.triwest.com/provider. Accessed on January 2, 2018.

[30] The Centers for Medicare and Medicaid Services manages the Medicare Exclusion Database (MED) which contains a list of excluded providers and their sanctions and reinstatement files. For additional information about the MED, see https://www.cms.gov/Research-Statistics-Data-and-Systems/Computer-Data-and-Systems/MED/Overview-MED.html. Accessed on January 2, 2018.

[31] To determine if a provider or entity is required to meet the Conditions of Participations (CoPs) and Conditions for Coverage (CfCs), see https://www.cms.gov/Regulations-andGuidance/Legislation/CFCsAndCoPs/index.html. Accessed on January 2, 2018.

After determining that a provider is eligible for participation, he or she may enroll (with Health Net and/or TriWest) as a VCP provider. At this time, the VA community care provider and respective third-party administrator (TPA) are to establish an agreed-upon reimbursement amount for rendered services to veterans. When Health Net or TriWest is unable to coordinate the delivery of health care services to veterans, local VA Medical Centers (VAMCs) may enter into VCP Provider Agreements with eligible VA community providers through the VAMCs Community Care Departments.[32]

Consults/Referral Processes[33]

Consults and referrals, known as the VA community care consults/referrals, are initiated in two different manners.[34] First, a VA physician may submit a VA community care consult/referral (through the Computerized Patient Record System [CPRS])[35] on behalf of a veteran when there is a clinical need for the veteran to receive timely medical services. Second, a veteran may request a VA community care consult/referral (from his or her VA provider or local VA staff) in order to receive a medical service that is also timely. Regardless of how the consult/referral is initiated, all VA community care consults/referrals are to be processed by the VA Community Care Coordination staff within the VA. VA community care consults/referrals are processed based on whether the veteran requires emergent or urgent care. For urgent VA community care consults/referrals,

---

[32] Veterans Choice Program (VCP) Provider Agreements may be authorized between local VA Medical Centers (VAMCs) and out-of-network VA community care providers only after Health Net or TriWest is unable to process a veteran's authorization request and/or schedule an appointment, within a timely manner, for the veteran.

[33] Major portions of this section are adapted from, Department of Veterans Affairs, Veterans Health Administration, VHA Chief Business Office, *Veterans Choice Program, Unusual or Excessive Burden Determination (Other Factors) Process*, December 2015.

[34] Generally, a veteran who becomes eligible under the VCP through the "30-day wait list" or "40 miles or more distance" pathway, may not have to go through the entire VA community care consult/referral process.

[35] The Computerized Patient Record System (CPRS) is the electronic system VA providers use to input consults/referrals for VA community care. Once entered, the VA community care consult/referral is to alert a clinical reviewer who is to examine the veteran's medical need and confirm that the requested services are not available at a local VA health care facility.

VA providers are to coordinate the veteran's care directly with the VA Community Care Coordination staff.

When a veteran's request for a VA community care consult/referral cannot be approved, the veteran's local VA facility staff are to notify the veteran. On behalf of the veteran, his or her VA provider is to continue coordinating the veteran's medical services within the VA. The veteran's provider might also explore other existing community care options (see *Table A-1*) offered by the Veterans Health Administration (VHA).

After a veteran's request is approved or the VA community care consult/referral is submitted by the veteran's provider, the VA Community Care Coordination staff are to confirm the veteran's eligibility status. A veteran may decline enrollment into the VCP. When a veteran declines enrollment, his or her respective third-party administrator (TPA) is to document the veteran's reason for opting out of the program. Then, on behalf of the veteran, his or her VA provider is to continue coordinating the veteran's medical services within the VA. The veteran's provider might also explore other existing community care options offered by the VHA.

If a veteran is found eligible to access care through the VCP, the VA Community Care Coordination staff is to then electronically upload the veteran's VA community care consult/referral and pertinent medical documentation in the Contractor Portal, which is visible to Health Net and TriWest. Once Health Net or TriWest receives the documentation, the respective TPA is to contact the veteran. During this contact, the eligible veteran is to be provided with an overview of VCP benefits and asked to confirm his or her choice to receive medical services under the VCP.

If a veteran reiterates his or her choice to receive medical care under the VCP, the veteran may select his or her VA community care provider and coordinate with a TPA to schedule an appointment. In addition, the veteran is to be asked to provide other health insurance information, if applicable, and is made aware of possible copayments and deductibles. A veteran with a clinical need for a service-connected and/or special authority condition[36]

---

[36] Special authority conditions include those that are eligible for service-connection under Priority Group 6 (combat veterans, ionization radiation, Agent Orange exposure, Southwest Asia

(SC/SA) is to have his or her screening information reviewed by Revenue Utilization Review (R-UR)[37] nurses. The veteran's appointment is then to be entered in the Contractor Portal so that it can be viewed by the VA Community Care Coordination staff. Daily, the VA Community Care Coordination staff is to check the Contractor Portal for appointment statuses and other updates. After the appointment is scheduled, the VA Community Care Coordination staff are to enter the appointment information into the Appointment Management system (within the VA) and update the veteran's status to "scheduled."

Unusual or Excessive Burden Determination[38]

Along with the environmental factors, geographic challenges, and medical conditions, veterans are assessed by

- the nature or simplicity of the hospital care or medical services the veteran requires,

---

service, veterans stationed at Camp Lejeune between August 1, 1953 to December 31, 1987, and Project 112/ SHAD), military sexual trauma, nasopharyngeal radium irradiation, etc.

[37] "R-UR, under the auspices of the CBO, is the systematic evaluation and analytical review of clinical information in order to maximize reimbursement from third-party payers. In 2003, guidance was established standardizing the clinical review functions with third-party reimbursement responsibilities at VA medical facilities. R-UR in this context operates to promote improvements in patient care and to maximize the potential for the recovery of funds due VA for the provision of health care services to Veterans, dependents, and others using the VA health care system." For more information, see Department of Veterans Affairs, Veterans Health Administration, *Utilization Management Program*, VHA Directive 1117, Washington, DC, July 9, 2014, p. 8, http://www.va.gov/vhapublications/ViewPublication. asp?pub_ID=3018. Accessed on January 2, 2018.

[38] Major portions of this section are adopted from Department of Veterans Affairs, Veterans Health Administration, VHA Chief Business Office, *Veterans Choice Program, Unusual or Excessive Burden Determination (Other Factors) Process*, December 2015. Also see, Department of Veterans Affairs, Veterans Health Administration, *Veterans Choice Program (VCP)*, Fact Sheet: Details on the Unusual or Excessive Burden Eligibility Criteria, May 27, 2017, https://www.va.gov/COMMUNITYCARE/docs/pubfiles/factsheets/VHA-FS_VCP-Eligibility.pdf. Accessed March 28, 2018.

- how frequently the veteran needs hospital care or medical services, and
- the need for an attendant for a clinical service.[39]

Authorization of Care and an Episode of Care

Prior to delivering medical services to veterans under the Veterans Choice Program (VCP), such services are to be authorized by the VA.[40] If a veteran requires services beyond those authorized, his or her VCP provider may request another authorization. The delivery and usage of unauthorized medical services could result in nonreimbursement. Under the VCP, over 2 million authorizations have been validated by the third-party administrators (TPAs) Health Net and

TriWest. These authorizations of care, shown in *Table 2*, were validated from November 5, 2014 to March 7, 2018, unless otherwise noted.

The VA defines an episode of care (EOC) as "a necessary course of treatment, including follow-up appointments and ancillary and specialty services, which last no longer than one calendar year from the date of the first appointment with a non-VA health care provider."[41] This one-year Choice EOC period of validity begins when the first appointment is scheduled. VA community care providers may request an authorization extension for a veteran's current EOC through the veteran's respective TPA.

---

[39] An attendant for clinical services is a person who provides essential aid and/or physical assistance to the veteran so that the veteran can travel to a VA medical facility to have hospital care or medical services rendered. 38 C.F.R. §17.1510(b)(4)(ii)(A)-(C).

[40] VA community care providers may call the Operation Center for Choice at (866) 606-8198 to request prior authorization from either Health Net or TriWest prior to delivering medical services to veterans. Failure to obtain preauthorization prior to rendering health services may result in uncompensated services.

[41] 38 C.F.R. §17.1505.

Table 2. Authorizations of Care for the Veterans Choice Program.
Mileage Eligibles and Wait-Time Eligibles from
November 2014 to March 7, 2018

	Health Net	TriWest	Totals
Unique Authorizations: Mileage Eligible[a]	186,362	362,998	549,360
Authorizations: Wait-Time Eligible	565,235	829,622	1,394,857
Authorizations: care is unavailable at the veterans' primary VA medical facility and cannot be referred to another VA facility (June 2015- March 7, 2018)[b]	887,199	1,402,949	2,290,148
Sub-Total Unique Authorizations: Wait-Time Eligible[c]	1,452,434	2,232,571	3,685,005
Total Authorizations	1,638,796	2,595,569	4,234,365

Source: Department of Veterans Affairs, Veterans Health Administration.

[a] Each authorization for an episode of care under this category is counted only once. One veteran patient could have more than one authorization.

[b] Based on the Department of Veterans Affairs, VA Care in the Community (Non-VA Purchased Care) and use of the Veterans Choice Program, Memorandum from Acting Principal Deputy Under Secretary for Health to Veterans Integrated Service Network (VISN) Directors, May 12, 2015, and amended on October 1, 2015, VA categorizes care that is unavailable at the veterans' primary medical facility and that cannot be referred to another VA facility or federal facility as care that would qualify for VCP under the wait-time eligible category.

[c] Each authorization for an episode of care under this category is counted only once. One veteran patient could have more than one authorization.

Appointment Scheduling

Veterans and VCP providers verify eligibility status before scheduling medical appointments for clinical needs. Appointments are to be scheduled on the basis of clinical appropriateness.[42] VCPeligible veterans are to receive a call from their respective third-party administrator (TPA), Health Net or TriWest. The TPAs are to provide veterans with information about the

---

[42] Ibid.

organization and schedule their appointments. Once appointments are scheduled, the contractor is to inform the VA. Emergent or urgent care authorizations are to be done expeditiously (see text box below).

Emergent and Urgent Care Determination

VA community care consults/referrals are to be prioritized by urgency levels. Urgency levels to deliver care are different under the VCP. Generally, emergent care under the VCP *does not* mean an emergency medical condition that needs immediate medical attention (emergency treatment furnished by non-VA providers are authorized under separate statutory authorities and not the VCP). Emergent consults/referrals are to be scheduled within five days from the veteran's consultation date with his or her third-party administrator (TPA). Urgent consults/referrals have a timeframe that is within 48 hours. Furthermore, VA providers may bypass the Choice Program process and contact the VA Community Care Coordination staff directly to schedule an urgent appointment with a VCP provider for their veterans.

After receiving the notification, a veteran's local VA facility staff are to cancel his or her appointment at the VA. Veterans may also choose to schedule their own appointments after receiving an authorization of care under the VCP.[43] If veterans choose to do so, they are asked to provide their appointment information to Health Net or TriWest.

Appointment information that is provided to the TPAs is to get uploaded into the Contractor's Portal, so that it can be viewed by the VA Community Care Coordination staff. Daily, the VA Community Care Coordination staff are to check the Contractor Portal for veterans' appointment statuses and other updates. After receiving the notification, the veteran's local VA facility staff are to cancel his/her appointment at the VA.

---

[43] Department of Veterans Affairs, "Expanded Access to Non-VA Care Through the Veterans Choice Program," 80 *Federal Register* 66424, October 29, 2015.

Medication Process

Veterans may have their prescriptions filled at their local VA pharmacies, non-VA pharmacies, and through the Consolidated Mail Outpatient Pharmacy (CMOP). If the VA is unable to fill a medication request within a prescribed timeframe or one that is not within the VA formulary, a non-VA pharmacy may fill the initial 14-day supply (without refills).[44] For veterans who require prescriptions for more than 14 days, the VCP prescribing clinician is to have the remaining supply of medication filled at a VA pharmacy. Similar to the provisions of health care services under the VCP, medications filled at non-VA pharmacies will also require prior authorizations from the VA.

The VA is to reimburse veterans for out-of-pocket expenses related to the purchase of medications that treat service-connected conditions. For nonservice-connected conditions, veterans may also be reimbursed for their out-of-pocket expenses, including those with other health insurance plans.[45] To be reimbursed, veterans submit a copy of their prescriptions, authorizations, and original receipts to their local VA Community Care Office. The VA also allows non-VA pharmacies to process medication claims on a veteran's behalf.

Processing Medical Claims

Medical claims under the Veterans Choice Program (VCP) are processed through the veteran's respective third-party administrators (TAPs). Health Net and TriWest upload and manage veterans' medical claims through the Contractors Portal. Through this web portal, the VA

---

[44] Veterans Health Administration, *Ten Things to Know About the Choice Program*, 2015, http://www.va.gov/HEALTH/newsfeatures/2015/July/10-Things-to-Know-About-Choice-Program.asp. Accessed on January 2, 2018.

[45] Department of Veterans Affairs, Veterans Health Administration, *Prescription Reimbursement Associated with VACC Delivered under the Choice Program*, VA Care in the Community (VACC) Program Reference Sheet, October 27, 2015. Department of Veterans Affairs, "Expanded Access to Non-VA Care Through the Veterans Choice Program," 79 *Federal Register* 65572, November 5, 2014.

Community Care Coordination staff are to retrieve a veteran's documentation of clinical need and upload it in the veteran's medical records.

The VA community care provider is to submit medical claims to a veteran's respective third-party administrator. After Health Net or TriWest receives the claim, the TPA is to submit it through its web portal. Subsequently, the VA is to retrieve the documentation from the TPA's web portal and upload it in the veteran's medical records. The VA reimburses the TPAs for the care veterans obtain through the VCP, and TPAs then reimburses the community care providers in their networks.[46]

> Per Federal authority, VA is the primary and exclusive payer for medical care it authorizes. As such, non-VA medical care providers may not bill the Veteran or any other party for any portion of the care authorized by VA. Federal law also prohibits payment by more than one Federal agency for the same episode of care; subsequently any payments made by the Veteran, Medicare, or any other Federal agency must be refunded to the payer [from the VCP provider] upon acceptance of VA payment.[47]

Medical Services Not Previously Authorized

Under the VCP, medical claims for unauthorized non-VA health care services may be submitted to the VA for payment consideration. Veterans, VA community care providers, and persons who paid for services on behalf of a veteran are required to submit to the VA the following documentation:

- a standard billing form,[48] or an invoice (i.e., Explanation of Benefits [EOB]), and/or receipt of services paid and/or owed;

---

[46] Department of Veterans Affairs, VA Office of Inspector General, Veterans Health Administration, Audit of Timeliness and Accuracy of Choice Payments Processed Through the Fee Basis Claims System, 15-03036-47, December 21, 2017, p. 6.

[47] Department of Veterans Affairs, Veterans Health Administration, Working with the Veterans Health Administration: A Guide for Providers, October 2014, p. 3, https://www.va.gov/COMMUNITYCARE/docs/pubfiles/programguides/ NVC_Providers_Guide.pdf. Accessed on January 2, 2018.

[48] The standard billing forms for reimbursement include the UB-04 CMS-1450 or CMS-1500.

- an explanation of the circumstance that led to the veteran receiving unauthorized care outside of the VA;
- any statements and/or supporting documentation;[49] *and*
- VA Form-10-583, Claim for Payment of Cost of Unauthorized Medical Services.[50]

PAYMENTS

Veterans' Out-of-Pocket Costs

Veterans who are enrolled in VA health care do not pay premiums,[51] deductibles,[52] or coinsurances[53] for their medical services. However, they may be required to pay a fixed copayment amount (for nonservice-connected disabilities or conditions) as shown below. When veterans receive care at a VA facility, they do not pay copayments at the time of their medical appointments; copayment rates are determined by the VA after services are furnished—based on if the care was for a service-connected or nonservice-connected condition. Therefore, veterans' out-of-pocket costs under the VCP are the same as if they were receiving care and services from a VA provider in a VA facility—if a veteran does not pay any copayments at VA health care facilities, the veteran will not have to pay any copayments under the VCP.[54] For example:

---

[49] 38 C.F.R. §17.124.
[50] VA Form 10-583, Claim for Payment of Cost of Unauthorized Medical Services, at http://www.va.gov/vaforms/form_detail.asp?FormNo=583. Accessed on January 2, 2018.
[51] An amount paid, by an enrollee or by an employer or a combination of both parties, to an insurer for a beneficiary to enroll in a health insurance plan.
[52] An amount a beneficiary must pay out of pocket before the health insurance plan begins paying for services.
[53] A specified percentage a beneficiary pays out of pocket to a provider after meeting any deductible requirements.
[54] Only veterans in Priority Group 1 (those who have been rated 50% or more service-connected) and veterans who are deemed catastrophically disabled by a VA provider are never charged a copayment, even for treatment of a nonservice connected condition. For more information, see Department of Veterans Affairs, "Criteria for a Catastrophically

- A veteran could pay $50 copayments for a specialty care visit and $15 for a primary care visit for a nonservice-connected disability or condition.
- A veteran in Priority Groups 2 thru 8 could pay a copayment between $5 and $11 per 30-day or less supply of medication.[55]
- All veterans are exempt from paying copayments for services and medications that are related to a service-connected disability or condition.[56]

Cost Shares for Veterans with Other Health Insurance (OHI)

The VA defines other health insurance (OHI) as commercial insurance. Commercial insurance, often referred to as *private insurance*, is not funded by federal and state taxes. This type of insurance is offered by companies such as Blue Cross and Blue Shield, Aetna, Cigna, and the Kaiser Foundation. Plans purchased through the state health exchanges are also considered as OHI. In addition, veterans who purchase commercial insurance plans agree to cost-sharing responsibilities. Such cost-sharing obligations include copayments, deductibles and coinsurance (e.g., 80/20 rule: 80% insurer responsibility/20% patient responsibility).

Due to various issues related to primary payment responsibility and veterans therefore experiencing adverse credit reporting to credit bureaus or debt collections by collections agencies, Congress enacted P.L. 115-26,

---

Disabled Determination for Purposes of Enrollment," 78 *Federal Register* 72576-72579, December 3, 2013.

[55] The VA categorizes veterans into eight Priority Groups, based on factors such as service-connected disabilities and income (among others). For a detailed summary of eight Priority Groups, see CRS Report R42747, *Health Care for Veterans: Answers to Frequently Asked Questions*, by Sidath Viranga Panangala.

[56] 38 C.F.R. §§17.108, 17.110, 17.111.

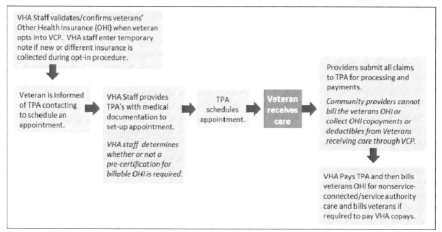

Source: Figure prepared by CRS based on information from the Veterans Health
      Administration.
Notes: VHA is Veterans Health Administration. TPA is Third-Party Administrators
      (Health Net Federal Services and TriWest Healthcare Alliance).

Figure 3. Coordination and Billing for Nonservice-Connected Care for Veterans with
Other Health Insurance (OHI). (This process is applicable to medical claims for all
services performed after April 19, 2017).

which amended P.L. 113-146 and made VA the primary payer for veterans
with OHI who seek care for nonservice-connected conditions through the
VCP. This change went into effect on April 19, 2017. The VA would
coordinate with a veteran's OHI and recover any costs, and bill the veteran
for any *copayments* that the veteran would be responsible for similar to what
they would have paid had they received care within a VA medical facility
(see *Figure 3*). Community care providers or the TPAs are no longer
required to collect copays, cost-shares, or deductibles from veterans with
OHI. Medicare, Medicaid, or TRICARE are not considered OHI plans under
the VCP.

Provider Payment Methodologies

Guidance on rates for the delivery of care is outlined in *Table 3*. As stated before, first, the Veterans Choice Program providers are to receive their reimbursements from either Health Net or TriWest. Then the VA is to reimburse the third-party administrator.[57] Eligible VA community care providers who decide to participate under the PC3 network (rather than the Choice network) may incur reimbursement rates lower than those of Medicare.[58] If these providers move to the Choice network, they may negotiate for a similar rate as contracted under the PC3 Network.

Veterans and VA community care providers may call the Community Care Call Center[59] to discuss billing issues. These issues range from the need to resolve a debt collection to inappropriately billed services.

Filing a Grievance with Health Net or TriWest[60]

Those veterans who have issues related to care provided by any of the two current TPAs (Health Net or TriWest) may file a grievance with their respective TPA. The grievance could be with regard to among other things, scheduling appointments, quality of care and services by the private network providers, and billing errors.[61]

---

[57] Department of Veterans Affairs, VA Office of Inspector General, Veterans Health Administration, Audit of Timeliness and Accuracy of Choice Payments Processed Through the Fee Basis Claims System, 15-03036-47, December 21, 2017, p. 6.

[58] Department of Veterans Affairs, "Expanded Access to Non-VA Care Through the Veterans Choice Program," 80 Federal Register 66425, October 29, 2015.

[59] Veterans may call the Community Call Center at 1-877-881-7618 from 9 am to 5 pm EST (https://www.va.gov/ HEALTHBENEFITS/cost/disputes.asp). Accessed on January 2, 2018.

[60] Department of Veterans Affairs, Veterans Health Administration, *Health Net and TriWest Complaint Process Patient-Centered Community Care (PC3) and Veterans Choice Program (VCP)*, February 15, 2018, https://www.va.gov/COMMUNITYCARE/docs/pubfiles/factsheets/VHA-FS_VACC-Complaint-Process.pdf. Accessed on March 28, 2018.

[61] Details on how to file a grievance is provided in, Department of Veterans Affairs, Veterans Health Administration, *Health Net and TriWest Complaint Process Patient-Centered Community Care (PC3) and Veterans Choice Program (VCP)*, February 15, 2018, https://www.va.gov/COMMUNITYCARE/docs/pubfiles/factsheets/VHA-FS_VACC-Complaint-Process.pdf. Accessed April 5, 2018.

Table 3. Payment Rates and Methodologies

	Episode of Care	
	Service-Connected Condition	Nonservice-Connected Condition
Payment Responsibilities	VA is solely responsible.	• VA is responsible for initial payment. The VA is required to then recover certain costs from the veterans Other Health Insurance (OHI)[a] • The veteran is responsible only for any copayments as required by the VA and not the veterans' OHI.
Payment Rates	Rates are not to exceed those in the "Medicare Fee Schedule;" with exceptions in highly rural areas, Alaska, All-Payer Model Agreements, and when there are no available rates.	
Highly Rural Areas[b]	• Higher rates that exceed the "Medicare Fee Schedule" may be negotiated.	
Alaska	• Rates are computed under 38 C.F.R. §§17.55(j), 17.56(b).	
All-Payer Model Agreements	• Rates are calculated based on the rates within the agreement.	
No Available Rates	• In this, the Secretary will follow the methodology outlined in 38 C.F.R. §§17.55, • 17.56.	
Authorized Care	Health Net or TriWest, on behalf of the VA, will authorize services.	
	The VA requires that all rendered services delivered to veterans receive prior-authorizations.	
	Medical services are delivered by an eligible entity or provider after a veteran chooses to receive care under the Veterans Choice Program.	

Source: 38 C.F.R. §17.1535.

[a] On April 19, 2017, P.L. 115-26 made the VA the primary payer for medical care provided for any nonservice-connected condition. The VA was required recover any costs from veterans' OHI plans. This removed the requirement that community providers and TPAs bill the veterans' OHI plans first.

[b] A "highly rural area" is defined as a county having fewer than seven individuals residing per square mile.

APPENDIX. VA CARE IN THE COMMUNITY

Table A-1 summarizes the existing major statutory authorities that allow the VA to provide care to veterans in the community utilizing non-VA providers.

Table A-1. VA Care in the Community.
Existing Statutory Authorities

Program Title	Description
Veterans' Choice Act (Veterans Choice Program) [38 U.S.C. §1701 note]	Temporary program, to furnish hospital care and medical services to eligible veterans through eligible VA community care providers. The program would expire whenever all the Veterans Choice Funds are expended.
Traditional VA Care in the Community (formerly Non-VA Medical Care or Fee- Basis Program) [38 U.S.C. §1703]	Authority to contract for hospital care and medical services when VA facilities are not capable of furnishing care due to geographic inaccessibility or are not capable of furnishing care; can also furnish counseling and related mental health services under 38 U.S.C. Section 1712A(e)(1).
Enhanced Sharing Authority [38 U.S.C. §8153]	Authority to make arrangement by contract or other forms of agreement, for the mutual use, or exchange of use, of health care resources between VA facilities and any health care provider, or other entity or individual. Sharing agreements with academic medical affiliates are executed under this authority.
Indian Health Service (IHS)/Tribal Health Program[a] (THP) [25 U.S.C §1645]	Authorizes the Secretary of Department of Health and Human Services (HHS) to enter into or expand sharing arrangements between IHS, tribes, and tribal organizations, and VA and Department of Defense (DOD).This authority is cited in VA's Direct Care Services reimbursement agreements with IHS and THP.
Sharing of VA and Department of Defense (DOD) Health Care Resources [38 U.S.C. §8111]	Authority to enter into sharing agreements and contracts with DOD for the mutual use or exchange of use of hospital and domiciliary facilities, and such supplies, equipment, material, and other resources as may be needed.
Emergency Care for Certain Veterans with Service-Connected Conditions[b] [38 U.S.C. §1728]	Authority to pay or reimburse charges of emergency treatment furnished in a non-VA facility where such treatment was needed for/related to a service-connected condition or in certain instances vocational rehab or provided to a veteran permanently and totally disabled.

Table A-1. (Continued)

Emergency Care for Nonservice-connected Conditions [38 U.S.C. §1725]	Authority to pay or reimburse charges of emergency treatment furnished in a non-VA facility under certain circumstances to certain eligible veterans.

Source: Table prepared by CRS based on U.S. Department of Veterans Affairs, Plan to Consolidate Programs of Department of Veterans Affairs to Improve Access to Care, October 30, 2015, pp. 104-107, http://www.va.gov/opa/ publications/VA_ Community_Care_Report_11_03_2015.pdf. Accessed on April 6, 2018.

Notes: This table does not show community care programs authorized under 38 U.S.C. §§1720 and 1720C, which includes community nursing home care, community adult health day care, home health care services, respite care, and hospice care.

[a] The VA and Indian Health Service/Tribal Health Programs signed a Memorandum of Understanding (MOU) to coordinate and share resources for services provided to eligible American Indian/Alaska Native Veterans.

[b] Treatment may be for either a service-connected condition or a nonservice-connected condition that is aggravating a service-connected connection.

In: The Veterans Choice Program (VCP)   ISBN: 978-1-53614-819-0
Editor: Mabel Page   © 2019 Nova Science Publishers, Inc.

Chapter 3

VETERANS CHOICE PROGRAM: IMPROVEMENTS NEEDED TO ADDRESS ACCESS-RELATED CHALLENGES AS VA PLANS CONSOLIDATION OF ITS COMMUNITY CARE PROGRAMS[*]

United States Government Accountability Office

ABBREVIATIONS

MRI	magnetic resonance imaging
PC3	patient-centered community care
REFDOC	referral documentation
RFP	request for proposals
TPA	third-party administrator
VA	Department of Veterans Affairs

---

[*] This is an edited, reformatted and augmented version of United States Government Accountability Office; Report to Congressional Addressees; Accessible Version, Publication No. GAO-18-281, dated June 2018.

VAMC   VA medical center
VHA   Veterans Health Administration
VISN   Veterans Integrated Service Network

WHY GAO DID THIS STUDY

Congress created the Choice Program in 2014 to address longstanding challenges with veterans' access to care at VHA medical facilities. The Joint Explanatory Statement for the Consolidated Appropriations Act, 2016 included provisions for GAO to review veterans' access to care through the Choice Program.

This chapter examines for Choice Program care (1) VA's appointment scheduling process, (2) the timeliness of appointments and the information VHA uses to monitor veterans' access; and (3) the factors that have adversely affected veterans' access and the steps VA and VHA have taken to address them for VA's future community care program.

GAO reviewed applicable laws and regulations, VA's TPA contracts, and relevant VHA policies and guidance. Absent reliable national data, GAO also selected 6 of 170 VAMCs (selected for variation in geographic location and the TPAs that served them) and manually reviewed a random, non-generalizable sample of 196 Choice Program authorizations. The authorizations were created for veterans who were referred to the program between January and April of 2016, the most recent period for which data were available when GAO began its review. The sample of authorizations included 55 for routine care, 53 for urgent care, and 88 that the TPAs returned without scheduling appointments. GAO also obtained the results of VHA's non-generalizable analysis of wait times for a nationwide sample of about 5,000 Choice Program authorizations that were created for selected services between July and September of 2016.

WHAT GAO RECOMMENDS

For VA's future consolidated community care program, GAO is making 10 recommendations, which include:

- establishing an achievable wait-time goal for the community care program that will permit VHA to monitor whether veterans are receiving care within time frames that are comparable to the amount of time they would otherwise wait for care at VHA medical facilities;
- designing an appointment scheduling process that (1) is consistent with the wait-time goal and (2) sets forth time frames within which veterans' referrals must be processed, appointments must be scheduled, and appointments must occur;
- implementing mechanisms to:
  - allow VHA to systematically monitor the amount of time taken to prepare referrals, schedule appointments, and complete appointments;
  - prevent veterans' clinically indicated dates from being modified by individuals other than VHA clinicians; and
  - separate clinically urgent referrals and authorizations from those for which the VAMC or the TPA has decided to expedite appointment scheduling for administrative reasons; and
- establishing a system that will help facilitate seamless, efficient care coordination and exchanges of information among VAMCs, VHA clinicians, TPAs, community providers, and veterans.

VA generally agreed with all but one of GAO's recommendations, which was to separate clinically urgent referrals from those that are administratively expedited. GAO maintains that implementing this recommendation will help improve future monitoring of urgent care timeliness for reasons explained in the report.

WHAT GAO FOUND

Through the Veterans Choice Program (Choice Program), eligible veterans may receive care from community providers when it is not readily accessible at Veterans' Health Administration (VHA) medical facilities. The Department of Veterans Affairs (VA) uses two contractors—or third party administrators (TPA)—to schedule most veterans' Choice Program appointments after receiving referrals from VA medical centers (VAMC). GAO found that veterans who are referred to the Choice Program for routine care because services are not available at VA in a timely manner could potentially wait up to 70 calendar days for care if VAMCs and the TPAs take the maximum amount of time VA allows to complete its appointment scheduling process. This is not consistent with the statutory requirement that veterans receive Choice Program care within 30 days of their clinically indicated date (when available), which is the soonest date that it would be appropriate for the veteran to receive care, according to a VHA clinician.

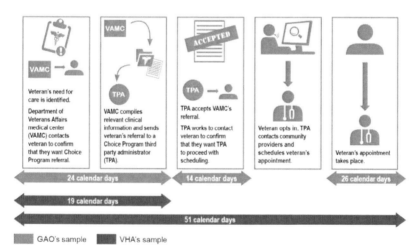

Source: GAO illustration based on GAO and VHA analyses of selected Choice Program authorizations. | GAO-18-281.

[a]GAO excluded from its analysis the amount of time the TPA took to schedule the appointment and the overall wait time because its sample selection methodology differed from VHA's in a way that would have skewed these two averages but not the averages for the other segments of the process.

Average Wait Times for Choice Program Appointments in 2016, According to Separate Non-Generalizable Analyses by GAO and the Veterans Health Administration (VHA).[a]

Without designing appointment scheduling processes that are consistent with this requirement, VA lacks assurance that veterans will receive Choice Program care in a timely manner.

GAO and VHA found that selected veterans experienced lengthy actual wait times for appointments in 2016, after manually reviewing separate samples of Choice Program authorizations. For example, when GAO analyzed 55 routine care authorizations that were created between January and April of 2016, it found that the process took at least 64 calendar days, on average. When VHA analyzed about 5,000 authorizations created between July and September of 2016, it took an average of 51 calendar days for veterans to receive care.

GAO also found that VHA cannot systematically monitor the timeliness of veterans' access to Choice Program care because it lacks complete, reliable data to do so. The data limitations GAO identified include:

- **A lack of data on the timeliness of referring and opting veterans in to the program.** GAO found that the data VHA uses to monitor the timeliness of Choice Program appointments do not capture the time it takes VAMCs to prepare veterans' referrals and send them to the TPAs, nor do they capture the time spent by the TPAs in accepting VAMCs' referrals and opting veterans in to the Choice Program. VHA has implemented an interim solution to monitor overall wait times that relies on VAMC staff consistently and accurately entering unique identification numbers on VHA clinicians' requests for care and on Choice Program referrals, a process that is prone to error.

- **Inaccuracy of clinically indicated dates.** GAO found that clinically indicated dates (which are used to measure the timeliness of care) are sometimes changed by VAMC staff before they send Choice Program referrals to the TPAs, which could mask veterans' true wait times. GAO found that VAMC staff entered later clinically indicated dates on referrals for about 23 percent of the 196 authorizations it reviewed. It is unclear if VAMC staff mistakenly entered incorrect dates manually, or if they inappropriately entered later dates when the VAMC was delayed in contacting the veteran, compiling relevant clinical information, and sending the referral to the TPA.

- **Unreliable data on the timeliness of urgent care.** GAO found that VAMCs and TPAs do not always categorize Choice Program referrals and authorizations in accordance with the contractual definition for urgent care. According to the contracts, a referral is to be marked as "urgent," and an appointment is to take place within 2 days of the TPA accepting it, when a VHA clinician has determined that the needed care is (1) essential to evaluate and stabilize the veteran's condition, and (2) if delayed would likely result in unacceptable morbidity or pain. GAO reviewed a sample of 53 urgent care authorizations and determined that about 28 percent of the authorizations were originally marked as routine care authorizations but were changed to urgent by VAMC or TPA staff, in an effort to administratively expedite appointment scheduling.

Without complete, reliable data, VHA cannot determine whether the Choice Program has helped to achieve the goal of alleviating veterans' wait times for care.

GAO found that numerous factors adversely affected veterans' access to care through the Choice Program. These factors include: (1) administrative burden caused by complexities of referral and appointment scheduling processes, (2) poor communication between VHA and its VAMCs, and (3) inadequacies in the networks of community providers established by the TPAs, including an insufficient number, mix, or geographic distribution of community providers. VA and VHA have taken numerous actions throughout the Choice Program's operation that were intended to help address these factors, though not all access factors have been fully resolved. For example, to help address administrative burden and improve the process of coordinating veterans' Choice Program care, VA established a secure e-mail system and a mechanism for TPAs and community providers to remotely access veterans' VA electronic health records. However, these mechanisms only facilitate a one-way transfer of necessary information. They do not provide a means by which VAMCs or veterans can view the TPAs' step-by-step progress in scheduling appointments or electronically receive medical documentation associated with Choice Program appointments.

While the Choice Program will soon end, VA anticipates that veterans will continue to receive community care under a similar program that VA plans to implement, which will consolidate the Choice Program and other VA community care programs. Incorporating lessons learned from the Choice Program into the implementation and administration of the new program could help VHA avoid similar challenges.

441 G St. N.W.
Washington, DC 20548

June 4, 2018

Congressional Addressees

The majority of veterans utilizing health care services delivered by the Veterans Health Administration (VHA) of the Department of Veterans Affairs (VA) receive care in VHA-operated medical facilities, including 170 VA medical centers (VAMC) and more than 1,000 outpatient facilities. In recent years, we and others have expressed concerns about the ability of VHA's medical facilities to provide health care services in a timely manner.[1]

---

[1] See, for example, GAO, *VA Health Care: Reliability of Reported Outpatient Medical Appointment Wait Times and Scheduling Oversight Need Improvement*, GAO-13-130 (Washington, D.C.: Dec. 21, 2012); GAO, *VA Health Care: Management and Oversight of Consult Process Need Improvement to Help Ensure Veterans Receive Timely Outpatient Specialty Care*, GAO-14-808 (Washington, D.C.: Sept. 30, 2014); GAO, *VA Primary Care: Improved Oversight Needed to Better Ensure Timely Access and Efficient Delivery of Care*, GAO-16-83 (Washington, D.C.: Oct. 8, 2015); and GAO, *VA Mental Health: Clearer Guidance on Access Policies and Wait-Time Data Needed*, GAO-16-24 (Washington, D.C.: Oct. 28, 2015). See also: Department of Veterans Affairs Office of Inspector General, *Healthcare Inspection: Gastroenterology Consult Delays, William Jennings Bryan Dorn VA Medical Center, Columbia, South Carolina*, Report No. 12-04631-313 (Washington, D.C.: Sept. 6, 2013) and Department of Veterans Affairs Office of Inspector General, *Veterans Health Administration, Review of Alleged Patient Deaths, Patient Wait Times, and Scheduling*

Serious and long-standing problems with veterans' access to care were also highlighted in a series of congressional hearings in the spring and summer of 2014, after several well-publicized events raised additional concerns about wait times for appointments at VHA medical facilities. In some cases, delays in care or VHA's failure to provide care reportedly have resulted in harm to veterans.[2] Due to these and other concerns, we concluded that VA health care is a high-risk area and added it to our High Risk List in 2015.[3]

In response to the problems with veterans' access to care at VHA medical facilities that were highlighted during the 2014 congressional hearings, Congress enacted the Veterans Access, Choice, and Accountability Act of 2014 (Choice Act) on August 7, 2014. Among other things, the law established a temporary program—called the Veterans Choice Program (Choice Program)—and provided up to $10 billion in funding for veterans to obtain health care services from non-VA community providers when they faced long wait times, lengthy travel distances, or other challenges accessing care at VHA medical facilities.[4] The temporary authority and funding for the Choice Program was separate from that of other previously existing programs through which VA has the option to purchase care from community providers. Legislation enacted in August and December of 2017 provided an additional $4.2 billion for the Veterans Choice Fund.[5] VA may continue to authorize Choice Program care until all amounts in the Choice Fund are exhausted.[6] Currently, VA is in the process

Practices at the Phoenix VA Health Care System, Report No. 14-02603-267 (Washington, D.C.: Aug. 26, 2014).

[2] See Department of Veterans Affairs Office of Inspector General, *Veterans Health Administration, Review of Alleged Patient Deaths, Patient Wait Times, and Scheduling Practices at the Phoenix VA Health Care System*.

[3] GAO, *High-Risk Series: An Update*, GAO-15-290 (Washington, D.C.: Feb. 11, 2015). GAO maintains a high-risk program to focus attention on government operations that it identifies as high risk due to their greater vulnerabilities to fraud, waste, abuse, and mismanagement or the need for transformation to address economy, efficiency, or effectiveness challenges.

[4] Pub. L. No. 113-146, §§ 101, 802, 128 Stat. 1754, 1755-1765, 1802-1803 (2014).

[5] VA Choice and Quality Employment Act of 2017, Pub. L. No. 115-46, § 101, 131 Stat. 958, 959 (Aug. 17, 2017) (providing an additional $2.1 billion for the Veterans Choice Fund); Department of Homeland Security Blue Campaign Authorization Act of 2017, Pub. L. No. 115-96. Div. D, § 4001, 131 Stat. 2044, 2052-53 (Dec. 22, 2017) (providing an additional $2.1 billion for the Veterans Choice Fund).

[6] Pub. L. No. 115-26, § 1,131 Stat. 129 (2017), amending section 101(p)(2) of the Choice Act, Pub. L. No. 113-146, 128 Stat. at 1763.

of planning its future community care program, which (as described in an October 2015 plan VA submitted to Congress) will consolidate the Choice Program and six other VA community care programs into one program.[7]

In accordance with the Choice Act, VA and VHA had up to 90 days to prepare for Choice Program implementation from the time the Choice Act was enacted. To cope with the compressed implementation time frame, VA modified contracts it had previously established with Health Net Federal Services (Health Net) and TriWest Healthcare Alliance (TriWest) to administer a different VA community care program and gave them certain responsibilities related to Choice Program administration, including the scheduling of routine and urgent care appointments for veterans needing care in the community.[8] VA and VHA refer to Health Net and TriWest as third-party administrators (TPA). The Choice Program implementation tasks included designing a framework to administer the program (which involved dividing responsibilities between VAMCs and TPAs), negotiating contract modifications to add Choice Program administration responsibilities to the TPAs' existing contracts with VA, designing referral and appointment scheduling processes for VAMCs and the TPAs, strengthening the community provider networks the TPAs had established under their existing VA contracts, creating TPA call centers, training VAMC and TPA staff,

---

[7] In this report, when we discuss VA's future community care program, we are referring to the plan for consolidating the Choice Program and VA's other community care programs that VA submitted to Congress on October 15, 2015. See Department of Veterans Affairs, *Plan to Consolidate Programs of Department of Veterans Affairs to Improve Access to Care*, (Washington, D.C.: Oct. 30, 2015). However, as of May 23, 2018, both Houses of Congress had passed S. 2371, the "VA Maintaining Internal Systems and Strengthening Integrated Outside Networks Act of 2018" (VA MISSION Act of 2018), which would establish a permanent community care program for veterans, among other purposes.

[8] Choice Program appointments that have not been categorized as "urgent" are considered to be appointments for routine care. Under VA's contracts with the TPAs, veterans' appointments are categorized as "urgent" when a clinician determines that the veteran needs care that (1) is considered essential to evaluate and stabilize conditions and (2) if not provided would likely result in unacceptable morbidity or pain when there is a significant delay in evaluation or treatment. Under VA's Choice Program contracts, urgent care is not the same as care provided for a medical emergency, which is covered through different VA community care programs. Urgent care (rather than emergent care) delivered through the Choice Program is care that is delivered when there is no threat to the veteran's life, limb, or vision but the veteran's condition needs attention to prevent it from becoming a serious risk to the veteran's health.

producing and distributing Veterans Choice Cards to veterans, and educating veterans and community providers about the new program.

External reviews, media reports, and congressional hearings held over the course of the Choice Program's implementation and operation have highlighted programmatic weaknesses, such as insufficient provider networks, significant delays in scheduling appointments, and a lack of timely payments to network providers.[9] The Joint Explanatory Statement for the Consolidated Appropriations Act, 2016 included two provisions for us to review veterans' access to care and the delivery of health care services through the Choice Program, with a focus on rural areas.[10] In addition, you asked us to conduct a comprehensive review of the Choice Program, focusing on (among other things) the effect the Choice Program has had on reducing veterans' wait times for care. In March 2017, we presented preliminary observations from this work at a hearing of the House Committee on Veterans' Affairs.[11]

This report updates our preliminary findings and examines:

1) the potential wait times for veterans to receive routine care through the Choice Program, according to VA's appointment scheduling process;

2) selected veterans' actual wait times to receive routine care and urgent care through the Choice Program and the information VHA uses to monitor access to care under the program; and

---

[9] See, for example, Department of Veterans Affairs Office of Inspector General, *Veterans Health Administration: Audit of the Timeliness and Accuracy of Choice Payments Processed Through the Fee Basis Claims System,* Report No. 15-03036-47 (Washington, D.C.: Dec. 21, 2017); Quil Lawrence, Eric Whitney, and Michael Tomsic, "Despite $10B 'Fix,' Veterans Are Waiting Even Longer To See Doctors." *Morning Edition* (radio program), May 16, 2016. Accessed January 27, 2017. http://www.npr.org/sections/health-shots/2016/05/16/477814218/attempted-fix-for-va-healt h-delays-creates-new-bureaucracy; and Lee Romney, "Veterans Choice is flawed, but Congress is stymied on a solution," *The Center for Investigative Reporting*, September 28, 2016. Accessed January 27, 2017. https://www.revealnews.org/article/veterans-choice-is-flawed-but-congress-is-stymied-ona-solution.

[10] 164 Cong. Rec. H10378, H10394 (daily ed. Dec. 17, 2015) (Explanatory Statement for Division J of the Consolidated Appropriations Act, 2016, Pub. L. No. 114-113 (2015)).

[11] See GAO, *Veterans' Health Care: Preliminary Observations on Veterans' Access to Choice Program Care,* GAO-17-397T (Washington, D.C.: March 7, 2017).

3) the factors, if any, that have adversely affected veterans' access to care under the Choice Program and the actions, if any, that VA and VHA have taken to address them for VA's future community care program.

To examine the potential wait times for veterans to receive routine care through the Choice Program according to VA's appointment scheduling process, we reviewed applicable laws and regulations; VA's contracts with the TPAs; and relevant VA and VHA policy directives, guidance, and training materials for VAMCs. In addition, we exchanged written correspondence with VA's Office of General Counsel about the application of VHA's wait time goals to the Choice Program. We also interviewed a VA contracting official and officials from VHA's Office of Community Care (the office responsible for implementing and overseeing the Choice Program), as well as officials from the two Choice Program TPAs, Health Net and TriWest.[12] We analyzed this evidence in the context of the federal internal control standard for control activities, which includes the design of policies and procedures that will help an entity achieve its objectives and respond to risks.[13]

To examine selected veterans' actual wait times to receive routine care and urgent care through the Choice Program and the information VHA uses to monitor access to care under the program, we took five key steps. We (1) analyzed Choice Program appointment wait times for selected veterans using a sample of 196 Choice Program authorizations for routine and urgent care; (2) reviewed VHA's analysis of appointment wait times for a sample of about 5,000 Choice Program authorizations; (3) reviewed data VHA uses

---

[12] Officials from VA's Denver Acquisition and Logistics Center are responsible for developing and managing Choice Program contracts with the TPAs. Contracting officer's representatives in VHA's Office of Community Care are responsible for monitoring the TPAs' performance. VHA's Office of Community Care is also responsible for developing policies and standard operating procedures, communicating contract modifications and other programmatic changes to VAMCs, and providing training for VAMC managers and staff on their roles in coordinating veterans' Choice Program care.

[13] See GAO, *Standards for Internal Control in the Federal Government*, GAO-14-704G (Washington, D.C.: Sept. 2014). Internal control is a process effected by an entity's oversight body, management, and other personnel that provides reasonable assurance that the objectives of an entity will be achieved.

to monitor the timeliness of Choice Program care and reasons that the TPAs have returned Choice Program referrals without making appointments; (4) interviewed VA, VHA, and TPA officials; and (5) reviewed federal internal control standards.[14] See Appendix I for more information on these methodological steps.

To examine the factors, if any, that have adversely affected veterans' access to care under the Choice Program and the actions, if any, that VA and VHA have taken to address them for VA's future community care program, we reviewed documentation and interviewed officials from VA, VHA, and the TPAs; as well as leadership officials and community care managers and staff from six selected VAMCs.[15] (See Appendix I for information about how we selected the six VAMCs.) In cases where we identified actions VA and VHA had taken to address factors that adversely affected veterans' access, we interviewed VA and VHA officials and reviewed documentation they provided to gain a better understanding of their rationale for taking those actions and the extent to which they had evaluated the outcomes or effectiveness of selected actions. Between May and September of 2016, we interviewed community care managers and staff at the six selected VAMCs, and we followed up with the managers in June and July of 2017. During these interviews, we discussed certain actions VA and VHA had taken and obtained their perspectives on implementation of the actions and the extent to which these actions improved veterans' access to Choice Program care. We examined the actions VA and VHA took in the context of federal standards for internal control.[16]

---

[14] For the Choice Program, the TPA generates an authorization after an eligible veteran has opted in to the program. Among other things, the authorization informs the community provider of the veteran's medical needs and the specific services that will be covered, as well as the period of validity (i.e., beginning and ending dates) for the episode of care. Each authorization may result in multiple appointments, and a single veteran may have multiple Choice Program authorizations.

[15] S. 2372, VA MISSION Act of 2018, was passed by both Houses of Congress after the completion of our audit fieldwork, and therefore, we did not incorporate it in our review of VA's future community care program. We evaluated the future community care program in light of the law current at the time of our audit and considering VA's 2015 plan for consolidating the Choice Program and VA's other community care programs, and tracked various legislative proposals for VA community care.

[16] GAO-14-704G.

We conducted this performance audit from April 2016 through May 2018 in accordance with generally accepted government accounting standards. Those standards require that we plan and perform the audit to obtain sufficient, appropriate evidence to provide a reasonable basis for our findings and conclusions based on our audit objectives. We believe that the evidence obtained provides a reasonable basis for our findings and conclusions based on our audit objectives.

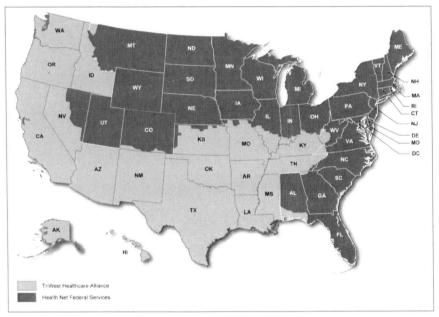

Sources: GAO illustration based on VHA information (data); Map Resources (map). | GAO-18-281.

Note: TriWest Healthcare Alliance is the TPA for American Samoa, Guam, and the Northern Mariana Islands. Health Net Federal Services is the TPA for Puerto Rico and the U.S. Virgin Islands.

Figure 1. Multi-state Regions Covered by the Veterans Choice Program's Third Party Administrators (TPA).

BACKGROUND

Responsibilities of the Choice Program TPAs

In October 2014, VA modified its existing contracts with two TPAs that were administering another VA community care program to add certain administrative responsibilities associated with the Choice Program. For the Choice Program, each of the two TPAs—Health Net and TriWest—is responsible for delivering care in a specific multi-state region (See Figure 1). Specifically, the TPAs are responsible for establishing networks of community providers, scheduling appointments with community providers for eligible veterans, and paying community providers for their services.

Choice Program Eligibility Criteria

As stated in VA's December 2015 guidance, the Choice Program allows eligible veterans to opt to obtain health care services from the TPAs' network providers rather than from VHA medical facilities when the veterans are enrolled in the VA health care system and meet any of the following criteria:[17]

- the next available medical appointment with a VHA clinician is more than 30 days from the veteran's preferred date or the date the veteran's physician determines he or she should be seen;
- the veteran lives more than 40 miles driving distance from the nearest VHA facility with a full-time primary care physician;
- the veteran needs to travel by air, boat, or ferry to the VHA facility that is closest to his or her home;

---

[17] Department of Veterans Affairs, Veterans Health Administration, *Veterans Choice Program Eligibility Details* (Washington, D.C.: Dec. 1, 2015).

- the veteran faces an unusual or excessive burden in traveling to a VHA facility based on geographic challenges, environmental factors, or a medical condition;[18]
- the veteran's specific health care needs, including the nature and frequency of care needed, warrants participation in the program;[19] or
- the veteran lives in a state or territory without a full-service VHA medical facility.[20]

Over the life of the Choice Program, VA has taken various approaches to care for veterans for whom services are not available at a particular VHA medical facility. In May and October of 2015, VHA issued policy memoranda to its VAMCs that required them to offer veterans referrals to the Choice Program before they authorized care through one of VA's other community care programs, which existed prior to the creation of the Choice Program.[21] Before May 2015, VA provided VAMCs the flexibility to decide on a case-by-case basis whether to refer veterans to the Choice Program or one of VA's other community care programs when services were not available. In June 2017, VHA issued another policy memorandum that rescinded the referral hierarchy that required VAMCs to refer to the Choice Program first. It directed VAMCs to refer veterans to the Choice Program only if they met the Choice Act's wait-time, distance, and geographic eligibility criteria, and to instead use other VHA medical facilities, facilities

---

[18] A determination about whether the veteran meets this criterion will be made in conjunction with staff at the veteran's local VHA medical facility.

[19] A determination about whether the veteran meets this criterion will be made in conjunction with staff at the veteran's local VHA medical facility.

[20] Specifically, veterans who reside in Alaska, Hawaii, New Hampshire, or a U.S. territory would be eligible for the program under this criterion. Veterans residing in New Hampshire are only eligible if they reside more than 20 miles away from the White River Junction VAMC, which is located in Vermont.

[21] See Veterans Health Administration, *VA Care in the Community (Non-VA Purchased Care) and Use of the Veterans Choice Program*, VHA Memoranda (May 12, 2015 and Oct. 1, 2015). Specifically, when services were unavailable or the veteran could not receive an appointment within 30 days, these memoranda required VAMCs to determine whether needed services are available in a timely manner from another VHA medical facility or from a facility with which the VAMC has a sharing agreement, such as a Department of Defense, Indian Health Service, or Tribal Health facility. If care could not be arranged in this manner, VAMCs had to offer eligible veterans the opportunity to receive care through the Choice Program before attempting to arrange care through any other VA community care program.

with which VA has sharing agreements, and other VA community care programs to deliver care to veterans when services were not available at a VHA medical facility and veterans did not qualify under the Choice Act's eligibility criteria. In August 2017, after Congress provided an additional $2.1 billion for the Choice Program, VHA again changed its guidance on referral patterns for the Choice Program and VA's other community care programs.[22] Specifically, VA issued a fact sheet saying that the new funding will allow VAMCs to refer veterans to the Choice Program to the maximum extent possible.[23] This allowed VAMCs to again offer veterans Choice Program referrals when services are unavailable at VHA medical facilities (until available funds have been exhausted), and also permitted VAMCs to refer veterans to other VA community care programs when services are unavailable.

Process for Choice Program Appointment Scheduling

Through policies and standard operating procedures for VAMCs and contracts with the TPAs, VA and VHA have established two separate processes for Choice Program routine and urgent appointment scheduling: one process for time-eligible veterans and another for distance-eligible veterans.[24]

Table 1 provides an overview of the appointment scheduling process that applies when a veteran is referred to the Choice Program because the veteran is time-eligible. (Appendix II contains additional detail about the Choice Program appointment scheduling process for time-eligible

---

[22] VA Choice and Quality Employment Act of 2017, Pub. L. No. 115-46, § 101, 131 Stat. 958, 959 (2017).

[23] See Department of Veterans Affairs, *Extension of Veterans Choice Program Funding,* VA Fact Sheet (August 2017).

[24] For the purposes of this report, the terms "time-eligible" and "distance-eligible" refer to the Choice Program processes used to schedule veterans' appointments. VHA uses the time-eligible appointment scheduling process when the services needed are not available at a VHA medical facility or are not available within allowable wait times. During this review, we did not evaluate VA's determination that veterans for whom services were unavailable were eligible for the Choice Program. VHA uses the distance-eligible appointment scheduling process when veterans reside more than 40 miles from a VHA medical facility or meet other travel-related criteria.

veterans—including differences between the routine and urgent care appointment scheduling process).

When veterans reside more than 40 miles from a VHA medical facility or meet other travel-related criteria, VHA uses the appointment scheduling process it developed for distance-eligible veterans. The process for distance-eligible veterans differs from that for time-eligible veterans in that VAMCs do not prepare a referral and send it to the TPA. Instead, distance-eligible veterans contact the TPA directly to request Choice Program care. See Table 2 for an overview of the Choice Program appointment scheduling process that applies for distance-eligible veterans. (See appendix III for additional detail about the Choice Program appointment scheduling process for distance-eligible veterans—including differences between the routine and urgent care appointment scheduling process).

Table 1. Process for Veterans to Obtain Department of Veterans Affairs (VA) Choice Program Care if They Are Time-eligible[a]

Steps of the Choice Program scheduling process	Completed by VA medical center (VAMC) staff	Completed by Choice Program third party administrator (TPA) staff	Completed by the veteran
A Veterans Health Administration (VHA) clinician determines the veteran needs care.	yes	n/a	n/a
VAMC staff confirm the veteran's eligibility for Choice Program care and begin contacting the veteran to offer a referral to the Choice Program.	yes	n/a	n/a
The veteran agrees to be referred to the Choice Program.	n/a	n/a	yes
VAMC staff compile relevant clinical information (including a description of the specific services and type of medical specialist the veteran needs) and submit the veteran's referral to the TPA.	yes	n/a	n/a

Table 1. (Continued)

Steps of the Choice Program scheduling process	Completed by VA medical center (VAMC) staff	Completed by Choice Program third party administrator (TPA) staff	Completed by the veteran
TPA staff review the veteran's Choice Program referral to ensure it contains information needed to proceed with appointment scheduling and accept the referral if the information is sufficient.	n/a	yes	n/a
TPA staff contact the veteran by telephone to confirm that they want to opt in to the Choice Program. If the veteran is not reached by telephone, the TPA sends a letter requesting that the veteran contact the TPA to opt in to the program.	n/a	yes	n/a
If the veteran opts in to the Choice Program, TPA staff create an authorization and begin efforts to schedule an appointment with a community provider.	n/a	yes	n/a
TPA staff schedule an appointment with a community provider. The authorization (which contains relevant clinical information, a description of authorized services, and a period of validity) is sent to the community provider. The veteran is informed of the date and time of the appointment.	n/a	yes	n/a
The veteran attends the initial appointment with the Choice Program community provider.	n/a	n/a	yes

Source: GAO analysis of VA and VHA documents. | GAO-18-281.

[a]VHA uses the time-eligible appointment scheduling process when the services needed are not available at a VHA medical facility or are not available within allowable wait times.

Table 2. Process for Veterans to Obtain Department of Veterans Affairs (VA) Choice Program Care if They Are Distance-eligible[a]

Steps of the Choice Program scheduling process	Completed by VA medical center (VAMC) staff	Completed by Choice Program third party administrator (TPA) staff	Completed by the veteran
The veteran contacts the TPA to request Choice Program care.	n/a	n/a	yes
TPA staff verify that the veteran is eligible for Choice Program care and that the requested care is medically appropriate.	n/a	yes	n/a
TPA staff create an authorization and begin efforts to schedule an appointment with a community provider.	n/a	yes	n/a
TPA staff schedule an appointment with a community provider. The authorization (which contains relevant clinical information, a description of authorized services, and a period of validity) is sent to the community provider. The veteran is informed of the date and time of the appointment.	n/a	yes	n/a
The veteran attends the initial appointment with the Choice Program community provider.	n/a	n/a	yes

Source: GAO analysis of VA and VHA documents. | GAO-18-281.

[a]VHA uses the distance-eligible appointment scheduling process when veterans reside more than 40 miles from a VHA medical facility or meet other travel-related eligibility criteria.

Choice Program Utilization from Fiscal Year 2015 through Fiscal Year 2016

Data we obtained from the TPAs indicate that VHA and the TPAs used the time-eligible appointment scheduling process about 90 percent of the time from fiscal year 2015 through fiscal year 2016 (the first 2 years of the Choice Program's implementation). More than half of the veterans who were referred to the Choice Program and for whom the TPAs scheduled appointments were referred because the services they needed were not available at a VHA medical facility.[25] The second-most-common reason for referral was that the wait time for an appointment at a VHA medical facility exceeded 30 days (See Figure 2). The distance-eligible appointment scheduling process was used for about 10 percent of the veterans who used the Choice Program between fiscal year 2015 through fiscal year 2016.

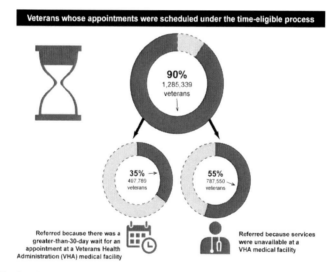

Figure 2. (Continued).

---

[25] Prior to obtaining these data from the TPAs, we requested data from VHA on the number of veterans who were referred to the Choice Program because (1) services were unavailable, (2) there was a greater than 30-day wait, or (3) the veteran resided more than 40 miles from a VHA facility or faced other travel burdens. However, VHA officials stated that VHA's data grouped veterans who were referred to the Choice Program because services were unavailable together with the veterans who were referred because of not meeting 30-day wait times. Only the TPAs could break these groups of veterans out separately, so we are instead reporting the TPAs' data.

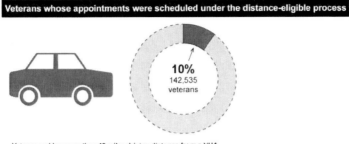

Veteran resides more than 40 miles driving distance from a VHA medicial facility or faces other travel burdens

Source: GAO analysis of data from Health Net Federal Services and TriWest Healthcare Alliance. | GAO-18-281.

Note: This excludes 7,198 veterans with scheduled appointments who were referred to the Choice Program in fiscal year 2015 and fiscal year 2016 because they faced an unusual or excessive travel burden to access care at a VHA medical facility. Only one of the two third party administrators (TPA) could separately report veterans who were referred under this Choice Program eligibility criterion. The other TPA does not distinguish veterans who were referred for unusual or excessive travel burden from the other three Choice Program referral reasons listed here.

Figure 2. Most Common Reasons Veterans with Scheduled Choice Program Appointments Were Referred to the Program, Fiscal Years 2015 through 2016.

Choice Act Wait-Time Requirements for Care Furnished under the Program

In coordinating the furnishing of care to eligible veterans under the Choice Program, VA is required to ensure that veterans receive appointments for Choice Program care within the wait-time goals of VHA for the furnishing of hospital care and medical services.[26] Although the Choice Act defined VHA's wait-time goals as not more than 30 days from the date a veteran requests an appointment from the Department, the Choice Act gave VA the authority to change this definition if it did not reflect VHA's actual wait-time goals. If VA wanted to exercise this authority, it was required to notify Congress of VHA's actual wait-time goals within 60

---

[26] Pub. L. No. 113-146, § 101(a)(3), 128 Stat. at 1756.

days of the law's enactment (i.e., by October 6, 2014).[27] VA did so in an October 3, 2014, report to Congress.[28] To "ensure that care provided through the Veterans Choice Program is delivered within clinically appropriate timeframes," VA notified Congress that VHA's wait-time goals were "not more than 30 days from either the date that an appointment is deemed clinically appropriate by a VA health care provider, or if no such clinical determination has been made, the date a Veteran prefers to be seen for hospital care or medical services." By incorporating VHA's reported wait-time goal, the Choice Act required VA to ensure the furnishing of care to eligible veterans within 30 days of the clinically indicated date or, if none existed, within 30 days of the veteran's preferred date.[29]

VA's Other Community Care Programs and Planned Consolidation

VA has purchased health care services from community providers through various programs since as early as 1945. Currently, there are six community care programs other than the Choice Program through which VA purchases hospital care and medical services for veterans. These six community care programs offer different types of services and have varying

---

[27] Pub. L. No.113-146, § 101(s), 128 Stat. at 1764.
[28] Department of Veterans Affairs, "Report to Congress on the Veterans Choice Program Authorized by Section 101 of the Veterans Access, Choice, and Accountability Act of 2014 (Pub. L. No. 113-146)," (Oct. 3, 2014). VA subsequently published the definition submitted to Congress in this report in the Federal Register, as required by section 101(s)(2)(B) of the Choice Act. See Department of Veterans Affairs: Wait-Time Goals of the Department for the Veterans Choice Program, 79 Fed. Reg. 62519-20 (October 17, 2014).
[29] The Choice Act's wait-time requirements apply to the furnishing of care to veterans who are eligible for the program under any of the Act's eligibility categories. Pub. L. No. 113- 146, § 101(a)(3), (b), (s)(2)(A), 128 Stat. at 1756-57, 1764. According to VHA policy, the clinically indicated date is the date that it would be clinically appropriate for the appointment to occur, as determined by the VHA clinician who identified the veteran's need for care. The clinically indicated date determination is based upon the needs of the patient and should be the soonest date that it would be clinically appropriate for the veteran to receive care. See Veterans Health Administration, *Consult Processes and Procedures,* VHA Directive 1232(1) (Aug. 24, 2016, as amended on Sept. 23, 2016).

eligibility criteria for veterans and community providers.[30] VA's six non-Choice community care programs include:

- **Individually authorized VA community care.** The primary means by which VHA has traditionally purchased community care is through individual authorizations, where local VAMC staff determine veteran eligibility, create authorizations, and assist veterans in arranging care with community providers that are willing to accept VA payment. Traditionally, VAMCs have approved the use of individually authorized community care when a veteran cannot access a particular specialty care service from a VHA medical facility because the service is not offered or the veteran would have to travel a long distance to obtain it from a VHA medical facility. (See appendix IV for an illustration of how appointment scheduling and care coordination processes for the Choice Program compare to those for individually authorized VA community care.)

- **Two emergency care programs.** When VA community care is not preauthorized, VA may reimburse community providers for emergency care under two different community care programs: 1) emergency care for a condition related to a veteran's service-connected disability and 2) emergency care for a condition not related to a veteran's service-connected disability, commonly referred to as Millennium Act emergency care.[31] For emergency care to be covered through these two programs, a number of criteria must be met, including (1) community providers must file claims in a timely manner (within 2 years of the date services were rendered for

---

[30] These six community care programs are the ones that VA proposed consolidating in the 2015 plan it submitted to Congress. See Department of Veterans Affairs, *Plan to Consolidate Programs of Department of Veterans Affairs to Improve Access to Care*. For more information about some of these VA community care programs, including differences in eligibility requirements and payment rates, see GAO, *Veterans' Health Care: Proper Plan Needed to Modernize System for Paying Community Providers,* GAO-16-353 (Washington, D.C.: May 11, 2016). There are other VA community care programs not described here—such as those that provide long-term care—that VA has not proposed including in its consolidation.

[31] The Veterans Millennium Health Care and Benefits Act, Pub. L. No. 106-117, § 111, 113 Stat. 1545, 1553-1556 (1999), codified, as amended, at 38 U.S.C. § 1725.

service-connected emergency care and within 90 days for Millennium Act emergency care); (2) the veteran's condition must meet the prudent layperson standard of an emergency; and (3) a VA or other federal medical facility must not have been feasibly available to provide the needed care, and an attempt to use either would not have been considered reasonable by a prudent layperson.[32]

- **Patient-Centered Community Care (PC3).** In September 2013, VA awarded contracts to Health Net and TriWest to develop regional networks of community providers to deliver specialty care, mental health care, limited emergency care, and maternity and limited newborn care when such care is not feasibly available from a VHA medical facility. VA and the TPAs began implementing the PC3 program in October 2013, and it was fully implemented nationwide as of April 2014—prior to the creation of the Choice Program. In August 2014, VA expanded the PC3 program to allow community providers of primary care to join the PC3 networks. PC3 is a program VA created under existing statutory authorities, not a program specifically designed by law. To be eligible to obtain care from PC3 providers, veterans must meet the same criteria that are required for individually authorized VA care in the community services.

---

[32] For both of VA's emergency care programs, a medical emergency exists when the condition is of such a nature that a prudent layperson would reasonably expect that delay in seeking immediate medical attention would be hazardous to life or health. The standard would be met if there was an emergency medical condition manifesting itself by acute symptoms of sufficient severity (including severe pain) that a prudent layperson who possesses an average knowledge of health and medicine could reasonably expect the absence of immediate medical attention to result in placing the health of the individual in serious jeopardy, serious impairment to bodily functions, or serious dysfunction of any bodily organ or part. See 38 C.F.R. § 17.1002(b) (2015). The prudent layperson standard emphasizes the patient's presenting symptoms, rather than the final diagnosis, when determining whether to pay emergency medical claims. The Millennium Act emergency care program has criteria in addition to those listed here that must be met in order for VA to pay claims from community providers. For more information about these criteria, see GAO, *VA Health Care: Actions Needed to Improve Administration and Oversight of VA's Millennium Act Emergency Care Benefit*, GAO-14-175 (Washington, D.C.: March 6, 2014).

- **Agreements with federal partners and academic affiliates.** When services are not available at VHA medical facilities, VA may also obtain specialty, inpatient, and outpatient health care services for veterans through two types of sharing agreements—those with other federal facilities (such as those operated by the Department of Defense and the Indian Health Service), and those with university-affiliated hospitals, medical schools, and practice groups (known as academic affiliates).

- **Dialysis contracts.** In June 2013, VA awarded contracts to numerous community providers nationwide to deliver dialysis—a life-saving medical procedure for patients with end-stage renal disease (permanent kidney failure). When dialysis services are not feasibly available at VHA medical facilities, veterans may be referred to one of VA's contracted dialysis providers, and veterans may receive dialysis at local clinics on an outpatient basis, or at home (if the contractors offer home-based dialysis services).

The VA Budget and Choice Improvement Act, which was enacted on July 31, 2015, required VA to develop a plan for consolidating all of its community care programs into a new, single program to be known as the "Veterans Choice Program."[33] VHA submitted this plan, including proposed legislative changes, to Congress on October 30, 2015. VA has moved forward with some aspects of the planned community care program consolidation that it believes can be accomplished without statutory changes. In December 2016, VA issued a request for proposals (RFP) for contractors to help administer the consolidated community care program, through "community care network" contracts. The consolidated community care program VA described in the October 2015 plan it submitted to Congress and the December 2016 RFP, as amended, would be similar to the current Choice Program in certain respects. For example, VA is planning to award community care network contracts to TPAs, which would establish regional networks of community providers and process payments to those

---

[33] Pub. L. No. 114-41, § 4002, 129 Stat. 443, 461 (2015).

providers. In contrast, other aspects of the consolidated community care program VA has planned may differ from the existing Choice Program. For example, VA's RFP for the community care network contracts, as amended, requires VAMCs—rather than TPAs—to carry out appointment scheduling, unless they exercise a contract option for the TPAs to provide such services.[34]

Annual Obligations for the Choice Program and Other VA Community Care Programs

Table 3. History of Annual Obligations for Health Care Services Provided Through the Veterans Choice Program (Choice Program) and Other Department of Veterans Affairs (VA) Community Care Programs

Obligations by fiscal year (in billions)			
Program	2015	2016	2017
Choice Program	$0.41	$1.50	$4.37
Other VA community care programs[a]	8.29[b]	7.49	6.79
Total	8.70	8.98	11.16

Source: GAO analysis of VHA data. | GAO-18-281

Note: The dollar figures in this table have been rounded to the nearest $10 million.

[a]Amounts in this row do not include obligations for VA-administered community care programs that serve veterans' dependents or family members, rather than veterans themselves. Such programs include the Civilian Health and Medical Program of the Department of Veterans Affairs, which is for family members of veterans who either (1) are rated by VA as permanently and totally or disabled, or (2) died from VA-rated service-connected disabilities. Also excluded from these amounts are obligations for VA's Primary Family Caregivers program and the Camp Lejeune Family Member Program because they also serve veterans' family members, rather than veterans.

[b]This amount includes $1.93 billion in Choice Program funds used by VA between May 1, 2015 and September 30, 2015 for other VA community care programs. Congress granted VA authority to use Choice Program funds for this purpose in July 2015. See Pub. L. No. 114-41, § 4004(a), 129 Stat. 443, 463 (2015). We have included these amounts as obligations of other VA community care programs because they were used for care through the other programs.

---

[34] A May 26, 2017 amendment to VA's December 2016 RFP gave VA the option of contracting with the TPAs to carry out the appointment scheduling process for VAMCs that request these services.

In fiscal year 2015, the first year of the Choice Program's implementation, total obligations for Choice Program health care services accounted for about 4.7 percent of the $8.7 billion VA obligated for all community care services that year.[35] However, as more care was provided through the Choice Program in fiscal years 2016 and 2017, obligations for Choice Program care grew steadily, while obligations for care delivered through other VA community care programs decreased. In fiscal year 2017, total obligations for Choice Program health care services accounted for about 39 percent of the $11.16 billion VA obligated for all community care services that year. See Table 3.

As shown in Table 4, below, of the $10.37 billion in Choice Program funds that were obligated between fiscal year 2015 and fiscal year 2017, $6.28 billion (or about 61 percent) of the funds were obligated for Choice Program health care services. About $1.76 billion (or 17 percent) of total Choice Program funds obligated between fiscal year 2015 and fiscal year 2017 were obligated for administrative costs. The remaining $2.33 billion (about 22 percent) were obligated for medical services other than those authorized under the Choice Program. As we previously reported, VHA experienced a projected funding gap in its medical services appropriation account in fiscal year 2015, largely due to lower-than-expected obligations for the Choice Program, higher-than-expected obligations for other VA community care programs, and unanticipated obligations for hepatitis C drugs.[36] To address the projected funding gap, on July 31, 2015, VA obtained temporary authority to use Choice Program funds between July 31, 2015 and September 30, 2015 for amounts obligated on or after May 1, 2015 to furnish

---

[35] An obligation is defined as a "definite commitment that creates a legal liability of the government for the payment of goods and services ordered or received, or a legal duty on the part of the United States that could mature into a legal liability by virtue of actions on the part of the other party beyond the control of the United States." GAO, *A Glossary of Terms Used in the Federal Budget Process*, GAO-05-734SP (Washington, D.C.: September 2005), p. 70.

[36] See GAO, *VA's Health Care Budget: In Response to a Projected Funding Gap in Fiscal Year 2015, VA Has Made Efforts to Better Manage Future Budgets,* GAO-16-584 (Washington, D.C.: Jun. 3, 2016). Prior to fiscal year 2017, VA's medical services appropriation funded VA health care services other than those authorized under the Choice Program—including services provided through VA's other community care programs. In fiscal year 2017, VA began funding non-Choice health care services through its annual medical services and medical community care appropriations, while services provided through the Choice Program were still funded through the Veterans Choice Fund.

medical services other than those that it authorized under the Choice Program. Later, in fiscal year 2016 and fiscal year 2017, VA de-obligated about $420 million of the Choice Program funds it had obligated for other VA community care programs and hepatitis C drugs in fiscal year 2015 because they were never expended.

Table 4. History of Veterans Health Administration (VHA)
Annual Obligations of Veterans Choice Program
(Choice Program) Funds, Fiscal Year 2015 through
Fiscal Year 2017

n/a	Amount of annual obligations, by fiscal year (in billions)			n/a
Obligation purpose	2015	2016	2017	Total obligations, fiscal year 2015 through fiscal year 2017 (in billions)
Choice Program health care services	$0.41	$1.50	$4.37	$6.28
Choice Program administration[a]	0.34	0.68	0.74	1.76
Other VA community care programs[b]	2.34	(.17)	(.23)	1.93
Hepatitis C drugs[b]	0.41	(.01)	—	.40
Total	3.50	2.0	4.87	10.37

Source: GAO analysis of VHA data. I GAO-18-281.

Note: The dollar figures in this table have been rounded to the nearest $10 million.

[a]These amounts include obligations for the implementation and administration of the Choice Program contracts as well as information technology support for the program.

[b]In fiscal year 2015, Congress authorized VHA to use Choice Program funds to address a projected funding gap of $2.75 billion, attributed to $2.34 billion in higher-than-expected obligations for VA's other community care programs and $0.41 billion in unanticipated obligations for hepatitis C drugs. Later, in fiscal year 2016 and fiscal year 2017, VA de-obligated about $0.42 billion of the Choice Program funds it had obligated for other VA community care programs and hepatitis C drugs in fiscal year 2015.

TIME ALLOWED TO COMPLETE VA'S CHOICE PROGRAM APPOINTMENT SCHEDULING PROCESS SIGNIFICANTLY EXCEEDS THE CHOICE ACT'S REQUIRED 30-DAY TIME FRAME FOR ROUTINE CARE

Our analysis of VA's scheduling process indicates that veterans who are referred to the Choice Program for routine care because they are time-eligible could potentially wait up to 70 calendar days to obtain care, if VAMCs and TPAs take the maximum amount of time allowed by VA's process.[37] About 90 percent of Choice Program referrals in fiscal years 2015 and 2016 were scheduled under the time-eligibility process, which means that the majority of veterans referred to the program would have been subject to this potential wait time for an appointment for routine care.[38] This 70-day potential wait time is in contrast to the Choice Act's required time frame, which is that eligible veterans receive Choice Program care no more than 30 days from the date an appointment is deemed clinically appropriate by a VHA clinician (referred to as the clinically indicated date), or if no such determination has been made, 30 days from the date the veteran prefers to receive care. According to VHA policy, a VHA clinician's clinically indicated date determination must be based upon the needs of the patient, and it should be the earliest date that it would be clinically appropriate for the veteran to receive care.[39] Therefore, if there is no clinical reason that care

---

[37] We updated our previous preliminary analysis of veterans' potential wait times, as reported in GAO-17-397T, because VA issued a relevant contract modification, guidance to the TPAs, and a VAMC policy memorandum after we testified before the Committee on Veterans' Affairs of the House of Representatives in March 2017. Previously, the overall potential wait time was 81 calendar days, but this contract modification, guidance, and policy memorandum reduced the overall potential wait time to 70 calendar days.

[38] In contrast, only about 10 percent of Choice Program authorizations created by the TPAs in fiscal years 2015 and 2016 were for distance-eligible veterans, which is why we did not separately examine potential wait times for these veterans. Under the TPA contracts, distance-eligible veterans are required to receive care within 30 days of their preferred dates, and they do not need to obtain referrals from VAMCs before contacting the TPAs to request appointments, which means that their overall wait times could potentially be less than 70 calendar days.

[39] See Veterans Health Administration, *Consult Processes and Procedures,* VHA Directive 1232(1) (Aug. 24, 2016, as amended on Sept. 23, 2016).

should be delayed, a veteran's clinically indicated date could be the same date that the VHA clinician determined the veteran needed care.[40]

The potential wait time of about 70 calendar days for time-eligible veterans to receive routine care through the Choice Program encompasses 18 or more calendar days for VAMCs to prepare veterans' Choice Program referrals and potentially another 52 calendar days for appointments to occur through the TPAs' scheduling process, as follows:

- **VAMCs' process for preparing routine Choice Program referrals.** According to VHA policies and guidance, VAMC staff have at least 18 calendar days to confirm that veterans want to be referred to the Choice Program and to send veterans' referrals to the TPAs:[41]
  - They have 2 business days (or up to 4 calendar days) after a VHA clinician has determined the veteran needs care to begin contacting an eligible veteran by telephone to offer them a referral to the Choice Program.
  - They have up to 14 calendar days after initiating contact to reach the veteran by telephone or letter and confirm that the veteran wants to be referred to the Choice Program.

[40] Among the sample of 196 Choice Program authorizations we reviewed, the clinically indicated date was the same date that the VHA clinician determined the veteran needed care about 60 percent of the time—in 82 out of the 134 authorizations for which we were able to identify clinically indicated dates. We could not identify VA's clinically indicated dates for a total of 62 of the authorizations in our sample. There were no clinically indicated dates for these 62 authorizations because (for example) they were for distance-eligible veterans who self-referred to the Choice Program or the authorizations were related to requests for additional services after veterans had already initiated an episode of Choice Program care.

[41] According to officials from VHA's Office of Community Care, VAMC staff are to follow VHA's policy directive for consult management when they are preparing veterans' Choice Program referrals. See Veterans Health Administration, *Consult Processes and Procedures,* VHA Directive 1232(1) (Aug. 24, 2016, as amended on Sept. 23, 2016) and a June 5, 2017 memorandum communicating new process timeliness scheduling requirements. VHA's Office of Community Care has provided further guidance related to the responsibilities of VAMC staff in preparing Choice Program referrals through standard operating procedures and training materials. The 18-calendar-day time period begins with the date the veteran's VHA clinician signaled the veteran's need for care by entering a consult into the veteran's VA electronic health record. A consult is a request entered by a VHA clinician on behalf of a patient seeking an opinion, advice, or expertise regarding evaluation or management of a specific problem.

- After confirming that a veteran wants to be referred to the Choice Program, however, VA has not set a limit on the number of days VAMCs should take to compile relevant clinical information and send referrals to the TPAs.

- **TPAs' process for scheduling routine Choice Program appointments.** Through its contracts with the TPAs, VA has established a process under which a veteran could potentially wait another 52 calendar days from the date the TPA receives the VAMC's Choice Program referral for a routine care appointment to take place. This includes up to 16 business days (or 22 calendar days) after receiving a referral to confirm the veteran's decision to opt in to the Choice Program and create an authorization. The contracts further state that, for time-eligible veterans, an appointment shall take place within 30 calendar days of the clinically indicated date, the authorization creation date, or the veteran's preferred date, whichever occurs later:

  - The TPA has 2 business days to review the VAMC's referral and accept it if it contains sufficient information to proceed with appointment scheduling.

  - The TPA has 4 business days to contact the veteran by telephone and confirm they want to opt in to the Choice Program (which means that the veteran wants to receive care through the Choice Program and have the TPA proceed with appointment scheduling).

  - If the veteran is not reached by telephone, the TPA has 10 business days for the veteran to respond to a letter confirming that they want to opt in, at which point the TPA creates the Choice Program authorization.

  - If the authorization is created after the veteran's preferred date or after the clinically indicated date on the VAMC's referral has already passed, the TPA has 30 calendar days from the authorization creation date for an appointment for routine care to take place.[42] The TPA can use up to 15 business days of this 30- calendar-day time frame to contact providers and successfully schedule the veteran's Choice Program appointment.[43]

See Figure 3 for an illustration of the potential wait time of approximately 70 calendar days for time-eligible veterans to receive routine care through the Choice Program.

The process VA established for time-eligible veterans to receive routine care through the Choice Program—which could potentially take 70 days to complete—is not consistent with the requirement that veterans receive care within 30 days of their clinically indicated dates (where available) as applicable under the Choice Act. Furthermore, according to the federal internal control standard for control activities, agencies should design control activities—such as through policies and procedures—that will help

---

[42] Among the sample of Choice Program authorizations we reviewed, the clinically indicated date had already passed before the TPA received the referral (and therefore before the authorization was created) in about 76 percent of the authorizations. This percentage is not surprising, given that VHA's consult policy directive instructs VHA clinicians to enter the earliest date an appointment is deemed clinically appropriate, which could be the same date that the veteran was first seen by the VHA clinician. Our 76 percent calculation is based on 134 of the 196 Choice Program authorizations in our sample. We could not identify either VA's clinically indicated date or the date the TPA received the referral for a total of 62 of the authorizations in our sample because (for example) the authorizations were for distance-eligible veterans who self-referred to the Choice Program or they were related to requests for additional services after veterans had already initiated an episode of Choice Program care. At the time the authorizations in our sample were created, time-eligible veterans' preferred dates were not taken into consideration by VA for the purposes of determining whether veterans' appointments for routine care occurred in a timely manner. Therefore, we could not determine what percentage of authorizations in our sample had preferred dates that had already passed before the TPA received the referral.

[43] Although the TPAs' contracts state that they must schedule veterans' appointments for routine care within 5 business days after the veterans opt in to the Choice Program or return the referrals to VAMCs if appointments have not been scheduled by the 10th business day, VA contracting officials sent a letter to the TPAs on June 15, 2017, to advise them of a temporary relaxation of that standard. Specifically, VA notified the TPAs that—until further notice—the TPAs will be allowed up to 15 business days to schedule appointments after veterans have opted in to the Choice Program and the TPAs have created authorizations. If appointments are not scheduled within 15 business days, the TPAs must return Choice Program referrals to the VAMCs so that they can attempt to arrange veterans' care through other means. According to VA contracting officials, they decided to relax the 5-day scheduling standard after the TPAs began returning a substantial volume of un-appointed referrals after the 10th business day, due to a variety of reasons that were outside the TPAs' control (such as community providers requesting additional medical documentation before agreeing to schedule appointments).

ensure federal programs meet their objectives and respond to any risks to meeting those objectives.[44]

A key reason that veterans' overall wait times for Choice Program care could potentially exceed the Choice Act's 30-day wait-time requirement is that the process VA and VHA designed did not include a limit on the number of days VAMCs have to complete a key step of the process— compiling relevant clinical information and sending referrals to the TPAs after veterans have agreed to be referred to the Choice Program. While the process sets forth time frames for the other steps VAMCs and TPAs must complete to process referrals and schedule appointments, VA and VHA have not specified how many days VAMCs have to send veterans' Choice Program referrals to the TPAs. VHA has no comprehensive policy directive for the Choice Program, and neither its consult management directive nor its outpatient appointment scheduling directive specifies an amount of time within which VAMCs should prepare Choice Program referrals.[45]

Another reason that veterans' overall wait times for Choice Program care could potentially exceed the Choice Act's 30-day wait-time requirement is that after VA and VHA implemented their policies, they did not review and address risks that were identified through their actual experience in operating the program. In response to a letter we sent in March 2017, VA's Deputy General Counsel for Legal Policy said that, based on VA's and VHA's experiences with actual operation of the Choice Program since November 2014, "the practical reality" has been that the 30-day wait-time goal VA established just prior to the program's implementation cannot always be met.

---

[44] GAO-14-704G.

[45] In October 2016, VHA issued a policy directive for the Choice Program, but it was not comprehensive because (among other things) it did not specify the number of days within which VAMCs' community care staff are required to send veterans' referrals to the TPAs after veterans have agreed to be referred to the Choice Program. See Veterans Health Administration, *Veterans Choice Program*, VHA Directive 1700 (Oct. 25, 2016). VHA's policy directive for consult management, which officials from VHA's Office of Community Care told us applies to the Choice Program, also does not specify this time frame. See Veterans Health Administration, *Consult Processes and Procedures*, VHA Directive 1232(1) (Aug. 24, 2016, as amended on Sept. 23, 2016).

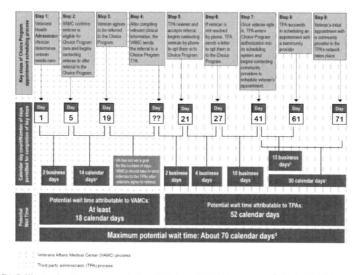

Source: GAO illustration based on analysis of VHA and TPA documents. | GAO-18-281.

Notes: This figure illustrates potential wait times for veterans who are referred to the Choice Program because VA determines they are time-eligible, if VAMCs and TPAs take the maximum amount of time allowed by VA's process. The terms "time-eligible" and "distance-eligible" refer to the Choice Program processes used to schedule veterans' appointments. VHA uses the time-eligible appointment scheduling process when the services needed are not available at a VHA medical facility or are not available within allowable wait times.

[a]VAMCs must attempt to contact veterans at least once by phone, and if the veterans are not reached, VAMCs must then send letters to the veterans and wait up to 14 calendar days for the veterans to respond that they want to be referred to the Choice Program.

[b]Although the TPAs' contracts state that they must schedule veterans' appointments for routine care within 5 business days after the veterans opt in to the Choice Program or return the referrals to VAMCs if appointments have not been scheduled by the 10th business day, VA contracting officials have temporarily relaxed that standard. Specifically, VA notified the TPAs via letter on June 15, 2017, that—until further notice—the TPAs will be allowed up to 15 business days to schedule appointments after veterans have opted in and the TPAs have created authorizations. If appointments are not scheduled within 15 business days, the TPAs must return Choice Program referrals to the VAMCs so that they can attempt to arrange veterans' care through other means.

[c]The 30-calendar-day appointment completion time frame begins with the date the TPA created the authorization only if the TPA creates the authorization for routine care after the clinically indicated date for a time-eligible veteran or the veteran's preferred date has already passed. Otherwise, appointments must occur within 30 calendar days of the clinically indicated date or the veteran's preferred date, whichever occurs later.

[d]The maximum potential wait time would be 68 calendar days if the veteran's need for care is identified on a Monday or Tuesday, and 70 calendar days if the veteran's need for care is identified on a Wednesday, Thursday, or Friday. If there are holidays, the total number of calendar days permitted to elapse may be greater than 68 or 70 calendar days.

Figure 3. Potential Wait Time for Time-Eligible Veterans to Obtain Routine Care through the Choice Program Appointment Scheduling Process.

VA has not disclosed what timeliness goals it would apply under a future consolidated community care program. We note, however, that VA currently has no timeliness goals for its existing individually authorized community care program and cannot determine the amount of time veterans wait, on average, to receive care through that program, which has accounted for a significant portion of veterans' community care utilization. We recommended in May 2013 that VA analyze the amount of time veterans wait to see providers in its individually authorized community care program and apply the same wait-time goals to that care that it uses to monitor wait times at VHA medical facilities.[46] VA concurred with the recommendation to conduct an analysis and reported that it was in the process of building wait-time indicators to measure wait-time performance for individually authorized VA community care. VHA has since updated its wait-time goal for care delivered within VHA medical facilities—which is that care must be delivered within 30 days of veterans' clinically indicated dates (where available). However, VA has not applied that same goal to its individually authorized VA community care program nor begun measuring wait-time performance for that program.

Timeliness of appointments is an essential component of quality health care; delays in care have been shown to negatively affect patients' morbidity, mortality, and quality of life. Without specifying wait-time goals that are achievable, and without designing appointment scheduling processes that are consistent with those goals, VA lacks assurance that veterans are receiving care from community providers in a timely manner. It also lacks a means for comparing the timeliness of veterans' community care with that of care delivered within VHA medical facilities.

---

[46] See GAO, *VA Health Care: Management and Oversight of Fee Basis Care Need Improvement,* GAO-13-441 (Washington, D.C.: May 31, 2013).

ACTUAL WAIT TIMES FOR CHOICE PROGRAM CARE HAVE BEEN LENGTHY FOR SELECTED VETERANS, AND VHA'S MONITORING OF VETERANS' ACCESS IS LIMITED BY INCOMPLETE AND UNRELIABLE DATA

In 2016, Selected Veterans Experienced Lengthy Overall Wait Times to Receive Routine Care and Urgent Care through the Choice Program

To examine selected veterans' actual wait times to receive routine care and urgent care through the Choice Program, we conducted a manual review of a random, non-generalizable sample of 196 Choice Program authorizations. The TPAs created these authorizations between January 2016 and April 2016 in response to referrals sent by six selected VAMCs.[47] Our manual review of veterans' VA electronic health records and the TPAs' records for our non-generalizable sample of 55 routine care authorizations and 53 urgent care authorizations for which the TPAs succeeded in scheduling appointments identified the following review times:

- For the 55 routine care authorizations in our sample, it took VAMC staff an average of 24 calendar days after the veterans' need for routine care was identified to contact the veterans and confirm that they wanted to be referred to the Choice Program, compile relevant clinical information, and send veterans' referrals to the TPAs. It

---

[47] The sample of authorizations we reviewed included only authorizations for which VHA's data indicated there were delays when the TPAs attempted to schedule appointments after the veterans had opted in to the program; however, our analysis of these authorizations indicates that delays occurred at other phases of the referral and appointment scheduling process as well. We found that many veterans in our sample experienced lengthy overall wait times for Choice Program care—as measured from the time their need for care was identified until they attended their initial appointments—and only a portion of the overall wait time could be explained by the TPA's delay in scheduling an appointment after the veteran opted in to the Choice Program.

took an average of 27 calendar days for the VAMCs to complete these actions for the 53 urgent care authorizations in our sample.[48]

- For these routine care authorizations, it took the TPAs an average of 14 calendar days to accept referrals and reach veterans by telephone or letter for the veterans to opt in to the Choice Program. It took the TPAs an average of 18 calendar days to complete these actions for the urgent care authorizations in our sample.

- After the TPAs succeeded in scheduling veterans' appointments for routine care, an average of 26 calendar days elapsed before veterans in our sample completed their initial appointments with Choice Program providers. For urgent care authorizations in our sample, it took an average of 18 days for the veterans to complete their initial appointments after the TPAs scheduled them.

See the following text box for specific examples of the overall wait times experienced by some veterans in the samples of routine and urgent Choice Program authorizations we reviewed.

Examples of Delays Experienced by Veterans for Whom the Choice Program Third Party Administrators (TPA) Scheduled Appointments

- One veteran was referred to the Choice Program for magnetic resonance imaging (MRI) of the neck and lower back because these services were unavailable at a Veterans Health Administration (VHA) medical facility. It took almost 3 weeks for Department of Veterans Affairs (VA) medical center (VAMC) staff to prepare his Choice Program referral for routine care and send it to the TPA, and then it took an additional 2 months after the VAMC sent the referral for the veteran to receive care. Notes in the veteran's VA electronic health record indicated that his follow-up

---

[48] We could not determine what portion of the total time it took VAMCs to prepare veterans' Choice Program referrals was accounted for by the interim steps of contacting the veteran or compiling relevant clinical documentation because we could not find in VA's electronic health record sufficient evidence of the dates these actions were completed for all of the authorizations in our sample.

appointment with a VHA neurosurgeon was at risk of being rescheduled because the VAMC had not received the results of the MRI after the appointment with the Choice Program provider occurred. Ultimately, the veteran's appointment with the VHA neurosurgeon—where the imaging results and treatment options were discussed—did not occur until almost 6 months after the VHA clinician originally identified the need for the MRI.

- One veteran was referred to the Choice Program because she needed maternity care, which is generally not available at VHA medical facilities. Almost a month and a half elapsed from the time VAMC staff confirmed her pregnancy (when she was 6 weeks pregnant) to when the VAMC sent the Choice Program referral for urgent care to the TPA. It then took 2 additional weeks for the TPA to make an unsuccessful attempt to contact the veteran to schedule a prenatal appointment; by that point, she was almost 15 weeks pregnant. The veteran called the TPA back, but when the TPA had yet to schedule an appointment by the time she was 18 weeks pregnant, the veteran finally scheduled her initial prenatal appointment herself, almost 3 months after her pregnancy was confirmed by VAMC staff.

- One veteran was referred to the Choice Program for thoracic surgery to address a growth on his lung because there was a wait for care at a VHA medical facility. TPA documentation we reviewed indicated that VAMC staff contacted the TPA four times to inquire about the status of the veteran's appointment, and the TPA contacted five Choice Program providers in its unsuccessful attempts to schedule the urgent appointment for the veteran. Ultimately, the veteran scheduled his own initial appointment with a thoracic surgeon in the community and informed the TPA that he had done so. The veteran's initial appointment occurred 3 weeks after the VAMC sent his referral to the TPA.

Source: GAO analysis of VHA and TPA documentation. | GAO-18-281.

Note: The above examples come from our random, non-generalizable sample of 55 authorizations for routine care and 53 authorizations for urgent care for which the Choice Program TPAs scheduled appointments between January 2016 and April 2016.

We also found that veterans in our sample experienced lengthy overall wait times to receive care when the TPAs returned their authorizations to the VAMC without scheduling appointments. When veterans' Choice Program authorizations are returned, VAMCs must attempt to arrange care through other means—such as through another VA community care program, a new Choice Program referral, or at another VHA medical facility. Among the 88 returned authorizations in our sample, we determined that 53 veterans eventually received care through other means after their authorizations were returned.[49] These 53 veterans ended up waiting an average of 111 days after the VHA clinician originally determined they needed care until their first appointment with a VHA clinician or with a community provider occurred. See the text box below for some examples of delays experienced by veterans in the sample of 88 returned Choice Program authorizations we reviewed.

Examples of Delays Experienced by Veterans Whose Authorizations Were Returned to Department of Veterans Affairs Medical Centers (VAMC) by the Choice Program Third Party Administrators (TPA)

The VAMC took almost 3 1/2 months to refer one veteran to a physical therapist to address her pelvic floor prolapse. When the preferred provider listed in the VAMC's referral was outside the TPA's network, the TPA sent a message to the VAMC via its web-based portal to ask if it should try scheduling the appointment with a different provider. By the time VAMC

---

[49] These 53 veterans received care either at a VHA medical facility, through another VA community care program, or through a new Choice Program authorization. We could not conclusively determine whether 20 of the 88 veterans in our sample received the care they needed after the TPAs returned their Choice Program authorizations. We provided these veterans' names to VHA officials in December 2016, and the officials followed up on these cases to ensure that the veterans got needed care and that patients were not harmed by any delay in care. In addition, 14 of the 88 veterans in our sample either declined care or no longer needed the care that was authorized. Three of those 14 veterans no longer needed care because they died before the TPAs or VAMCs could schedule appointments. Determining whether veterans in our sample experienced clinical harm or adverse clinical outcomes because of delays in the VAMCs' or TPAs' processing of their referrals and authorizations was outside the scope of our review; however, VHA officials with clinical expertise reviewed these cases and concluded that the patients' deaths did not result from any delay in care. The one remaining veteran in our sample was no longer eligible for services, which is why the TPA returned her authorization to VA.

staff responded to the message in the TPA's portal, the TPA had already returned the authorization—almost 2 weeks after accepting it. Two months later, the VAMC realized that the veteran still needed this care and sent a new Choice Program referral to the TPA. It then took the veteran another 2 1/2 months to attend her first appointment. Overall, this veteran waited more than 8 months to receive physical therapy.

- One veteran who was eligible for the Choice Program because he resided more than 40 miles from a VHA medical facility contacted the TPA to request an appointment with a urologist. More than a month later, the TPA contacted the VAMC via its web-based portal to request a referral for the veteran. VAMC staff responded to the TPA two days later and stated (correctly) that because the veteran was distance-eligible, no referral was required. Four days after receiving the VAMC's response, the TPA succeeded in scheduling an appointment.
  However, the veteran declined it because the TPA had scheduled the appointment with a neurologist (a specialist who treats conditions affecting the brain, spinal cord, and nerves) rather than a urologist (a specialist who treats conditions affecting the urinary tract and male reproductive organs). Ultimately, the veteran ended up seeing a urologist at a VAMC nearly 5 months after he originally contacted the TPA to request care.
- It took about 2 1/2 weeks for the VAMC to send one veteran's referral for pain management to the TPA after a VHA clinician originally determined he needed these services. However, information the TPA needed for scheduling the Choice Program appointment was missing from the VAMC's referral. The TPA requested the information from the VAMC twice using its web-based portal, but VAMC staff did not reply, and the TPA returned the authorization 2 weeks after receiving it. It then took another month before the veteran ended up receiving pain management services at a VAMC. Overall, this veteran waited almost 2 1/2 months for pain management services.

Source: GAO analysis of VHA and TPA documentation. | GAO-18-281.

Note: The above examples come from our random, non-generalizable sample of 88 Choice Program authorizations that the TPAs returned to six VAMCs between January 2016 and April 2016.

After we shared the results of our preliminary analysis with VHA officials in December 2016, VHA required its medical facilities to manually review a sample of about 5,000 Choice Program authorizations that were created in July, August, and September of 2016 for four types of Choice Program care—mammography, gastroenterology, cardiology, and neurology. The purpose of this review was to analyze (1) the timeliness with which VAMCs sent referrals to the TPAs, and (2) veterans' overall wait times for Choice Program care. VHA calculated the average wait imes across these four types of care for each of its 18 Veterans Integrated Service Networks (VISN).[50]

VHA's analysis of data collected by VAMCs identified the following average review times when veterans were referred to the Choice Program because there was a greater-than-30-day wait time for an appointment at a VHA medical facility.

- **Referral wait times.** VISN-level averages ranged from 6 to 53 days for VAMC staff to contact veterans and confirm that they wanted to be referred to the Choice Program, compile relevant clinical information, and send veterans' referrals to the TPAs. The national average was 19 days.
- **Overall wait times.** From the time veterans' need for care was identified until they attended initial Choice Program appointments, average overall wait times ranged from 34 to 91 days across VHA's 18 VISNs. The national average was 51 days.

When veterans were referred to the Choice Program because services were unavailable at a VHA medical facility, VHA's analysis of VAMCs' self-reported data identified the following average review times:

---

[50] VHA's health care system is divided into areas called VISNs, each responsible for managing and overseeing medical facilities within a defined geographic area. VISNs oversee the day-to-day functions of VA medical facilities that are within their boundaries. Currently, there are 18 VISNs nationwide.

- **Referral wait times.** VISN-level averages ranged from 6 to 21 days for VAMC staff to contact veterans and confirm that they wanted to be referred to the Choice Program, compile relevant clinical information, and send veterans' referrals to the TPAs. The national average was 15 days.
- **Overall wait times.** From the time veterans' need for care was identified until they attended initial Choice Program appointments, average overall wait times ranged from 39 to 56 days across VHA's 18 VISNs. The national average was 47 days.

VHA's Monitoring of Veterans' Access to Choice Program Care Is Limited by a Lack of Complete, Reliable Data

Our analysis indicates that VHA's ability to monitor Choice Program access is limited because the data VHA uses are not always accurate and reliable, and VHA lacks certain data that are needed to effectively monitor the program. As discussed below, multiple factors contribute to these data limitations. According to federal internal control standards for information and communication and for monitoring, agencies should use quality information to achieve the entity's objectives, internally and externally communicate quality information, and establish activities to monitor the quality of performance over time and evaluate the results.[51] Without complete, reliable Choice Program data, VHA cannot determine whether the Choice Program has achieved the goals of (1) alleviating the wait times veterans have experienced when seeking care at VHA medical facilities, and (2) easing geographic burdens veterans may face to access care at VHA medical facilities.

---

[51] GAO-14-704G.

VHA Cannot Systematically Calculate the Average Number of Days VAMCs Take to Prepare Choice Program Referrals

The data VHA currently uses to monitor the timeliness of Choice Program appointment scheduling and completion do not capture the days it takes for VAMCs to prepare veterans' referrals and send them to the TPAs. This is because VHA has not standardized the manner in which VHA clinicians and VAMC staff categorize consults that lead to Choice Program referrals.[52]

We observed inconsistency in the titles of consults that were associated with the non-generalizable sample of Choice Program authorizations we reviewed. For example,

- consult titles sometimes included the word "Choice," but in other cases they included the words "non-VA care."
- Some of the consult titles indicated the criterion under which the veteran was eligible for the Choice Program and the type of care the veteran needed (for example, "Choice-First Physical Therapy"), while other consult titles only indicated the type of care the veteran needed (for example, "pain management").[53]

We observed this variability among consult titles both within single VAMCs and across all six of the VAMCs we selected for review.

According to documentation VHA officials provided to us in December 2016, they planned on implementing a process for standardizing the consult

---

[52] A consult is an electronic request entered in VA's electronic health record by a VHA clinician who is seeking an opinion, advice, or expertise regarding evaluation or management of a veteran's condition. For the purposes of the Choice Program, the consult entry date is the date a veteran's need for care was originally identified. When there is a wait for an appointment at a VHA medical facility, staff at the VAMC use information from the consult—such as the clinically indicated date determined by the VHA clinician and a description of needed services—to prepare veterans' Choice Program referrals.

[53] The term "Choice-First" pertains to veterans who are referred to the Choice Program because services are unavailable at a VHA medical facility or the veteran cannot receive an appointment at a VHA medical facility or another federal medical facility within VHA's timeliness standards. It comes from VHA's May and October 2015 policy memoranda, which required VAMCs to offer eligible veterans the opportunity to receive care through the Choice Program before attempting to arrange care through any other VA community care program.

titles associated with Choice Program referrals over the course of calendar year 2017. Originally, they planned on piloting the process at four VAMCs beginning in February 2017 and expected to gradually roll out standardized consult titles across all other VAMCs over the remainder of calendar year 2017. However, in late June and early July 2017, we followed up with the six VAMCs in our sample, and at that time, managers from only one of the VAMCs said that they had implemented the new process for standardizing consult titles associated with Choice Program referrals. When we interviewed VHA officials again in September 2017, they acknowledged that they had been delayed in implementing standardized consult titles, and they provided documentation indicating that they were just beginning to roll out the new process nationwide.

In the absence of standardized consult titles for the Choice Program, VHA has no automated way to electronically extract data from VA's electronic health record and calculate the average number of days it takes for VAMC staff to prepare veterans' Choice Program referrals after veterans have agreed to be referred to the program. Further, without standardized consult titles, VHA cannot monitor veterans' overall wait times—from the time VHA clinicians determine veterans need care until the veterans attend their first appointments with Choice Program providers. The lack of standardized consult titles also prevents VHA from tracking average overall wait times and monitoring the timeliness of care for veterans whose Choice Program authorizations are returned by the TPAs without scheduled appointments.

Available VHA Data Do Not Capture the Time Spent by TPAs in Accepting VAMCs' Referrals and Opting Veterans in to the Choice Program

The data VHA currently uses to monitor the timeliness of Choice Program appointments capture only a portion of the process that the TPAs carry out to schedule veterans' appointments after they receive referrals from VAMCs. Specifically, VHA's data reflect the timeliness of appointment scheduling and completion after the TPAs create authorizations in their appointment scheduling systems, which (according to VA's contracts, as of June 1, 2016) the TPAs must do only after they have received all necessary information from VA and the veteran has opted in to the Choice Program. Therefore, VHA's timeliness data do not capture the time TPAs spend (1) reviewing and accepting VAMCs' referrals, and (2) contacting veterans to confirm that they want to opt in to the Choice Program.

- **Data related to the timeliness of Choice Program appointment scheduling.** When we asked how they monitor the timeliness of Choice Program appointment scheduling, VHA officials provided us the following types of data, all of which reflect the time that elapses only after veterans have opted in to the Choice Program and the TPAs have created authorizations:
  - the average number of business days the TPAs take after creating authorizations to schedule appointments for routine and urgent care,
  - the percentage of appointments for routine care that the TPAs schedule within 5 business days after they create authorizations, and
  - the percentage of appointments for urgent care that the TPAs schedule within 2 business days after they create authorizations.
- **Data related to the timeliness with which initial Choice Program appointments occur.** VHA officials provided us data on the timeliness with which initial Choice Program appointments have occurred; however, as shown below, almost all of these data reflect the timeliness with which appointments occur only after veterans have opted in to the Choice Program and the TPAs have either created authorizations or successfully scheduled veterans' appointments:
  - the average number of business days after the TPAs create authorizations in which appointments for routine and urgent care occur;
  - the percentage of appointments for routine care that are completed within 30, 60, 90, and 120 business days or more after the TPAs create an authorization;

- the percentage of appointments for routine care that are completed within 30 calendar days of either (1) the TPA's scheduling of the appointment, (2) the clinically indicated date on the VAMC's referral, or (3) the veteran's preferred date; and
- the percentage of appointments for urgent care that are completed within 2 calendar days of the TPAs creating the authorizations.

See Figure 4 for an illustration of how VHA's data capture only a portion of the Choice Program process to obtain care.

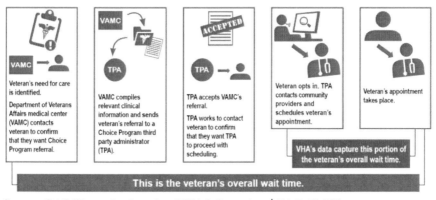

Source: GAO illustration based on VHA information. | GAO-18-281.

Figure 4. Illustration of How the Veterans Health Administration's (VHA) Data Capture Only a Portion of the Choice Program Process for Obtaining Care.

In September 2017, VHA officials told us that they recently began implementing an interim solution that would allow them to track veterans' overall wait times for Choice Program and other VA community care— from the time VHA clinicians determine veterans need the care until the veterans attend their first appointments with community providers. Specifically, this interim solution requires VAMC staff to enter unique identification numbers on VHA clinicians' requests for care and on the Choice Program referrals they send to the TPAs. This unique identification number is then carried over to the Choice Program authorizations that are created in the TPAs' systems. According to VHA officials, the unique identification number creates a link between VHA's data and the TPAs' data, so that VHA can monitor the timeliness of each step of the Choice Program referral and appointment scheduling process. However, the success of VHA's interim solution relies on VAMC staff consistently and accurately entering the unique identification numbers on both the VHA clinicians' requests for care and on Choice Program referrals, a process that is prone to error. VHA officials said it is their long-term goal to automate the process by which VHA's data are linked with TPAs' data in the consolidated community care program they are planning to implement.

Because, as previously explained, VHA lacks data on the average timeliness with which VAMCs prepare Choice Program referrals, and VHA also lacks data on the average amount of time that elapses between when the TPAs receive VAMCs' referrals and when veterans opt in with the TPAs, VHA cannot track veterans' overall wait times for Choice Program care—from the time VHA clinicians determine that veterans need care until the veterans attend their first appointments with Choice Program providers. In addition, the lack of data on the timeliness with which the TPAs have (1) accepted VAMCs' referrals and (2) determined that veterans wish to opt in to the program also prevents VHA from assessing whether the TPAs' average timeliness in completing these actions has improved over time.

Clinically Indicated Dates Are Sometimes Changed by VAMC Staff Before They Send Choice Program Referrals to the TPAs

Our analysis of a sample of 196 Choice Program authorizations shows that another way in which VHA's monitoring of veterans' access to care is limited by available data is that the clinically indicated dates included on referrals that VAMCs send to the TPAs may not be accurate. We found that the clinically indicated dates on VAMCs' referrals were not always identical to the clinically indicated dates that were originally entered into VA's electronic health record by the VHA clinicians who treated the veterans.

VHA's policy directive on consult management and its Choice Program standard operating procedure for VAMCs state that the clinically indicated date is to be determined by the VHA clinician who is treating the veteran. However, in reviewing VA's electronic health records for our sample of 196

Choice Program authorizations, we identified 60 cases where the clinically indicated dates VAMC staff entered on Choice Program referrals they sent to the TPAs differed from the clinically indicated dates that were originally entered by VHA clinicians.[54] In 46 of these 60 cases, VAMC staff entered clinically indicated dates on the Choice Program referrals that were later than the dates originally determined by the VHA clinicians, which would make the veterans' wait times appear to be shorter than they actually were.

VHA could not explain why the dates differed. Clinically indicated dates are manually entered on VAMCs' electronic referrals to the TPAs, a practice that is subject to error or manipulation. It is unclear if VAMC staff mistakenly entered incorrect dates, or if they inappropriately entered later dates when the VAMC was delayed in contacting the veteran, compiling relevant clinical information, and sending the referral to the TPA. If VAMCs' Choice Program referrals have clinically indicated dates that are different from the ones VHA clinicians originally entered without additional supporting documentation, there is a risk that VHA's data will not accurately reflect veterans' actual wait times. Specifically, VHA will not be able to determine how often veterans receive Choice Program care within the Choice Act's required 30-day time frame.

VAMCs and TPAs Frequently Re-Categorize Routine Choice Program Referrals as Urgent Referrals, Sometimes Inappropriately

Another limitation of VHA's monitoring of veterans' access to Choice Program care is that VAMCs and TPAs do not always categorize referrals in accordance with the contractual definition for urgent care when they are processing referrals and scheduling appointments for veterans. According to VA's contracts with the TPAs, Choice Program referrals are to be marked as "urgent" when a VHA clinician has determined that the veteran needs care that (1) is considered essential to evaluate and stabilize conditions and

---

[54] We were able to identify clinically indicated dates for 134 of the 196 Choice Program authorizations in our sample. We could not identify VA's clinically indicated dates for a total of 62 of the authorizations in our sample. There were no clinically indicated dates for these 62 authorizations because (for example) they were for distance-eligible veterans who self-referred to the Choice Program or the authorizations were related to requests for additional services after veterans had already initiated an episode of Choice Program care.

(2) if not provided would likely result in unacceptable morbidity or pain when there is a significant delay in evaluation or treatment.[55] It is VA's goal that the TPAs schedule appointments for urgent care and ensure that they take place within 2 business days of accepting the referrals from VA.

Among the sample of 53 Choice Program authorizations for urgent care we reviewed, VHA and TPA documentation showed that in 35 cases (about 66 percent), VHA clinicians originally determined that veterans needed routine care, but VAMC or TPA staff later re-categorized the referrals or authorizations as urgent. In 4 of these 35 cases, we found documentation showing that VHA clinicians had reviewed the pending referrals and determined that the veterans' clinical conditions or diagnoses warranted re-categorizing the veterans' routine care referrals or authorizations as urgent.[56] In 31 other cases we reviewed, however, we found no documentation indicating that a VHA clinician had identified a clinical reason for the veteran to receive care faster. In at least 15 of these 31 cases, it appeared that the VAMC or TPA staff changed the status of the referral or authorization in an effort to administratively expedite appointment scheduling when they were delayed in sending referrals and scheduling veterans' Choice Program appointments.

According to the VA contracting officer who is responsible for the Choice Program contracts, VA's contracts with the TPAs do not include provisions for separating clinically urgent Choice Program referrals and authorizations from those that the VAMC or the TPA has decided to expedite for administrative reasons (such as when the veteran or VAMC staff has expressed frustration with a delay in the referral or appointment scheduling process). If Choice Program referrals for routine care are inappropriately categorized as urgent care referrals under the Choice Program, VHA's data on the timeliness of urgent appointment scheduling

---

[55] Under VA's Choice Program contracts, urgent care is not the same as care provided for a medical emergency, which is covered through different VA community care programs. Urgent care (rather than emergent care) delivered through the Choice Program is care that is delivered when there is no threat to the veteran's life, limb, or vision but the veteran's condition needs attention to prevent it from becoming a serious risk to the veteran's health.

[56] Determining whether veterans in our sample experienced clinical harm or adverse clinical outcomes because of delays in the VAMCs' or TPAs' processing of their referrals and authorizations was outside the scope of our review.

and completion will not accurately reflect the extent to which veterans who have a clinical need for urgent care are receiving it within the time frames required by the TPAs' contracts.

The TPAs' Choice Program Performance Data Did Not Become Comparable until 18 Months after the Program Began, Which Limits VA's Ability to Monitor Whether Access Has Improved

The authorization creation date is the primary starting point from which VHA monitors the TPAs' timeliness in appointment scheduling and the extent to which veterans' initial Choice Program appointments occur in a timely manner. However, when initially implementing the Choice Program—beginning in November 2014—the two TPAs had differing interpretations of contractual requirements relating to when they should create authorizations in their appointment scheduling systems. According to VA contracting officials and VHA community care officials we interviewed, at the start of the program, one of the TPAs was creating authorizations as soon as it accepted referrals from VAMCs, but the other was waiting until after veterans opted in to the Choice Program to create authorizations. It was not until May 2016 (about 18 months into the Choice Program's implementation) that VA modified its contracts to clarify that the TPAs are to create Choice Program authorizations only after they have contacted the veterans and confirmed that they want to opt in to the program.

Due to these differing interpretations, VA lacked comparable performance data for the two TPAs for the first 18 months of the Choice Program's expected three-year implementation. Therefore, it could not compare the timeliness of access nationwide. In addition, since VA modified the TPAs' contracts midway through the Choice Program's implementation, officials can only comparatively examine whether the timeliness of both TPAs' appointment scheduling and completion has improved since June 2016, which is when the relevant contract modification took effect.

TPAs Sometimes Select Incorrect Return Reasons or Inappropriately Return Choice Program Authorizations without Making Appointments

VHA collects data and monitors various reasons the TPAs return Choice Program authorizations to VAMCs without making appointments.[57] Each month, VA monitors how each TPA performs on Choice Program performance measures related to the timeliness of appointment scheduling. Authorizations that are returned for reasons that are attributable to the TPA—such as a lack of network providers in close proximity to the veteran's residence—negatively impact the TPAs' monthly performance measures.

In our sample, we found that VHA's data on the TPAs' reasons for returning Choice Program authorizations are not reliable. Specifically, we questioned the validity of the TPAs' return of 20 out of the 88 authorizations in our sample, for the following reasons:

- In 11 of the 20 cases, we found VHA or TPA documentation that substantiated the return, but the TPAs selected the incorrect return reasons when they sent the authorizations back to VA. For example, in one case, the TPA was unable to schedule an appointment with a primary care provider—even after contacting 11 different network providers—but the TPA staff returned the authorization to the VAMC indicating that the veteran had declined care. TPA officials who reviewed this authorization with us agreed that it was inappropriate to mark this authorization as having been returned because the veteran declined care and that their staff instead should have indicated that they had been unable to schedule an appointment with a network provider.

---

[57] VA has established through its contracts a set of acceptable reasons for the TPAs to return Choice Program authorizations without making appointments. Among other things, VA monitors the percentage of authorizations that the TPAs returned because (1) VAMCs' referrals were missing information the TPAs needed to schedule appointments, (2) the TPA was unable to reach a network provider who would schedule an appointment and see the veteran, (3) the veteran rejected the appointment because the time or location the TPA offered was inconvenient, or (4) the veteran decided they no longer wanted to receive care through the Choice Program.

- In the remaining 9 of the 20 cases, we could find no VHA or TPA documentation to substantiate the reasons the TPAs selected when they returned the authorizations to VA, nor any other reasons for return. For example, the TPAs incorrectly selected "missing VA data" as the reason they returned 5 of these 9 authorizations. Based on VHA and TPA documentation we reviewed, the VAMCs' referrals were complete and not missing any of the information the TPAs needed to proceed with appointment scheduling.

TPA officials could not explain why their staff selected incorrect return reasons or inappropriately returned authorizations for which they should have kept attempting to schedule appointments. However, TPA staff must manually select return reasons when they send authorizations back to VAMCs, a process that is subject to error or manipulation. There is a process by which VA's contracting officer's representatives validate the monthly data submitted by the TPAs, but it cannot identify the data reliability issues we found when manually reviewing VHA and TPA documentation associated with a sample of returned Choice Program authorizations. VHA officials told us that VA's contracting officer's representatives do not have access to veterans' electronic health records, which means that they cannot check whether VHA documentation substantiates the return reasons selected by the TPAs.

Without reliable data on reasons that veterans have been unable to obtain appointments through the Choice Program, VHA cannot properly target its efforts to address challenges—such as network inadequacy— that may be causing the TPAs to return authorizations without making appointments.[58] In addition, the lack of reliable data makes it difficult for VA to monitor whether the TPAs are meeting their contractual obligations, such as establishing adequate networks of community providers.

---

[58] Network adequacy relates to the number, mix, and geographic distribution of community providers that participate in the TPA's network.

VHA Does Not Have Performance Measures for Monitoring Average Driving Times between Veterans' Homes and the TPAs' Choice Program Network Providers

Another way in which VHA's monitoring of veterans' access is limited is that VA lacks contract performance measures that would provide VA and VHA with data related to veterans' driving times to access care from the TPAs' Choice Program network providers. Such performance measures would help VA monitor the TPAs' network adequacy. In contrast, for PC3, VA does collect data from the TPAs to monitor urban, rural, and highly rural veterans' maximum commute times to specialty care providers, providers of higher level care, primary care providers, and mammography and maternity care providers.

When we asked why VA had not established driving time performance measures for the Choice Program, a VHA official responsible for monitoring the Choice Program contracts told us he thought that these performance measures had simply been overlooked in the haste to implement the Choice Program. VA concurred with a recommendation we made in our December 2016 report about VA health care for women veterans, in which (among other things) we stated that the department should monitor women veterans' driving times to access sex-specific care through the Choice Program and VA's future community care contracts.[59] However, VA stated in its June and October 2017 written updates on actions it has taken to address this recommendation that it does not intend to modify the current Choice Program contracts to address our recommendation because the contracts will be ending soon and it would be too costly to do so. Without driving time performance measures for the Choice Program, VHA lacks assurance that the TPAs' networks include a sufficient number of community providers in close proximity to where veterans live, and it cannot monitor the extent to which veterans' geographic access to care has improved or diminished.

---

[59] See GAO, *VA Health Care: Improved Monitoring Needed for Effective Oversight of Care for Women Veterans*, GAO-17-52 (Washington, D.C.: December 2, 2016).

MULTIPLE FACTORS HAVE ADVERSELY AFFECTED VETERANS' ACCESS TO CARE UNDER THE CHOICE PROGRAM, PROVIDING POTENTIAL LESSONS LEARNED FOR VA'S FUTURE COMMUNITY CARE PROGRAM

Officials we interviewed from VA's contracting office, VHA's Office of Community Care, and both of the TPAs, along with leadership officials, managers, and staff from the six selected VAMCs told us about various factors that have directly or indirectly affected veterans' access to care throughout the Choice Program's implementation. Chief among these are (1) administrative burden associated with the Choice Program's complex referral and appointment scheduling processes; (2) inadequate VAMC staffing and poor communication between VHA and the VAMCs; and (3) the TPAs' slow development of a robust provider network. We also identified actions VA and VHA have taken to address these factors. (See appendix VI for additional information about actions that VA and VHA took to address these three access-related issues for the Choice Program.) To the extent that these factors persist under the consolidated community care program that VA plans to establish, they will continue to adversely affect veterans' access to care.

VA and VHA Took Several Actions to Address Administrative Burden Caused by Complex Choice Program Processes, but Opportunities Still Exist to Improve Care Coordination

VHA and TPA officials, as well as managers and staff from the six selected VAMCs, told us they encountered administrative burden associated with the complexities of the Choice Program's referral and appointment scheduling processes. Further, they lacked care coordination tools throughout the time they were operating the Choice Program, which affected their ability to provide timely care to veterans.[60] Among the main issues cited were the following:

- **Manual referral processes and lack of TPA access to veterans' records.** To prepare veterans' Choice Program referrals, VAMC staff had to follow a manual, time-consuming process to retrieve and collate key contact and clinical information from veterans' VA electronic health records. This was because—throughout most of the Choice Program's implementation—VA had no system for automatically generating referral packages that contained all of this information; nor did TPA staff have access to veterans' VA electronic health records. If VAMC staff made mistakes (such as mistyping or inadvertently omitting veterans' telephone numbers or addresses) or if the referrals were missing clinical information that the TPAs needed for appointment scheduling purposes, the TPAs had to either contact the VAMC to correct or obtain the missing information or return the referrals to VA without attempting to schedule appointments. These manual processes impeded the VAMCs' progress in preparing referrals and the TPAs' progress in scheduling veterans' Choice Program appointments.

- **Limited availability of care coordination tools and dependence on telephone-based customer service for appointment scheduling.** A lack of care coordination tools and near-constant telephone calls also delayed VAMC and TPA staff from efficiently processing veterans' referrals for appointments. For example, the Choice Program had no web-based portal through which VAMC staff and veterans could view the TPAs' step-by-step progress in scheduling appointments. While both of the TPAs had portals that

---

[60] The Agency for Healthcare Research and Quality defines care coordination as the practice of organizing patient care activities and sharing information among all of the participants concerned with a patient's care to achieve safer, more effective care. Participants may share clinical data using manual methods such as faxing paper records, but these methods can be time-consuming and costly. Information technology has the potential to improve the efficiency of care coordination by allowing VA, the TPAs, community providers, and veterans to electronically exchange information for care coordination purposes.

allowed VAMC staff (but not veterans) to obtain certain information— such as whether the TPA had already scheduled an appointment—the portals did not show if, or when, veterans' referrals had been accepted, the dates and times of the TPAs' attempts to contact veterans, or the number of community providers the TPA had contacted in its attempts to schedule an appointment. VAMC staff we interviewed said that while they could submit written messages to the TPAs through the portals, TPA staff did not always answer these messages in a timely manner. This, in turn, made telephone calls between veterans, the VAMCs, and the TPAs the most effective form of follow-up regarding veterans' Choice Program referrals, according to VAMC managers and staff. Officials from one selected VAMC estimated that their community care staff (which included about 30 employees) was answering approximately 10,000 calls per month, and another VAMC had hired a full-time staff person just to answer telephone calls.

- **Workload associated with re-authorizing veterans' care.** VAMC and TPA staff also told us they faced a lengthy administrative process to re-authorize care if veterans' Choice Program authorizations expired before veterans received care or if veterans needed services that were outside the scope of their original authorizations. The TPAs referred to these as "secondary authorization requests" or "requests for additional services." Without these re-authorizations, veterans' care from community providers could be delayed or interrupted.[61] VAMC and TPA staff had to process a high volume of these requests for two main reasons. First, the Choice Program originally had a 60- day limit on episodes of care, which meant that all appointments within the episode of care had to be completed within 60 days of the initial date of service. Even if the veteran needed care that could routinely be expected to outlast this 60-day time frame (such as maternity care or cancer

---

[61] The high volume of re-authorizations also indirectly affected the timeliness of other veterans' access to Choice Program care because it diverted VAMC and TPA staffs' attention from processing other veterans' referrals and scheduling appointments.

treatment), community providers and the TPAs would still have to request additional referrals from the VAMCs to authorize the remaining care. Second, TPAs would have to request additional referrals if an episode of Choice Program care was already in progress and the veteran needed services that were not specifically authorized in the VAMC's original referral. According to some VAMC managers and staff, this generated significant workload for the VAMCs. Officials from one of the selected VAMCs said it had to hire a full-time nurse just to process secondary authorization requests.

- **Manual post-appointment follow-up processes.** According to VAMC managers and staff we interviewed, the manual processes used for post-appointment follow-up also added to delays for veterans seeking care through the Choice Program. After an episode of care is complete—whether services are delivered at a VHA medical facility or in the community—VHA's policy requires VAMC staff to document that care was provided and make the results of encounters available to VHA clinicians by entering medical records or other clinical information into the veteran's VA electronic health record.[62] When medical records from the community provider became available, VAMC staff had to retrieve copies from the TPAs' portals and scan them into veterans' VA electronic health records. (See appendix V for an illustration of this process.) VAMC staff described this as a very time-consuming ...cess because it could take months for claims or medical records ...ice Program appointments to appear in the TPAs' portals. ... our interviews in the summer of 2016, managers from ... in our sample said they each had backlogs of ... Program and other community care ... backlog adversely affected veterans' ... because the time VAMC staff spent

Consult... es and Procedures, VHA Directive ...on Sept. 2...).

attempting to complete some veterans' consults could not be spent on preparing other veterans' Choice Program referrals.

Over the course of the Choice Program's implementation, VA and VHA took multiple actions to address administrative burden, including the following. Opportunities exist to improve or build on these actions as VA moves forward with the consolidated community care program it plans to implement.

- **Implementation of a web-based tool to automate Choice Program referral preparation.** In early 2016, to improve the process of gathering information from veterans' VA electronic health records to prepare Choice Program referrals, staff from two VAMCs developed a web-based tool—called the "referral documentation" (REFDOC) tool. According to VHA documentation, the REFDOC tool automates the process of gathering necessary information and assembling it in a standardized format for veterans' Choice Program referrals. VHA's initial analyses of the REFDOC tool's effectiveness found that it sped up the process of preparing Choice Program referrals by about 20 minutes per referral, which helped reduce the administrative burden associated with preparing referrals. However, VHA's nationwide dissemination of the tool to all of the VAMCs was slowed by limitations of VA's information technology systems. As of November 2016 (about 9 months after the tool was created), it had only been implemented at 18 of VHA's 170 VAMCs. VH gradually made the tool available at the remaining VAMCs betw November 2016 and May 201.

- **Standardized episodes of care.** In April 2017, VHA a' standardized episodes of care—"bundles" of clinically medical services and procedure that are to be whenever veterans are referred community p specified types of care. This w intended to administrative burden associated with nical revie improve veterans' access to care. To start, VHA approved standardized episodes of care for 15 different types of care, including physical therapy, maternity care, and optometry. VA and VHA documentation indicate that they intend to roll out additional standardized episodes of care over time and continue using them once VA transitions to the consolidated community care program it is planning to implement.

- Acquisition of a secure e-mail system and a mechanism for TPAs and community providers to remotely access veterans' VA electronic health records. VA recently established two different care coordination tools that were intended to make the process of providing veterans' medical records to Choice Program and other VA community care providers more efficient.

  - *Secure e-mail system.* In the spring of 2017, VA acquired software that allows VAMC managers and staff to e-mail encrypted files containing veterans' medical records to the TPAs and community providers. Only the intended recipient can decrypt and respond to messages containing the files. According to VHA documentation, this secure e-mail system was intended to improve the efficiency of coordinating veterans' Choice Program care and address potential security risks associated with printing paper copies of veterans' medical records and sending them to the TPAs or community providers via fax or U.S. mail.

  - *Remote access to veterans' VA electronic health records.* In May 2017, VHA began offering a secure, web-based application called the Community Viewer as a tool for community providers nationwide to have access to assigned veterans' VA electronic health records. Like the secure e-mail system, this tool is intended to improve the efficiency of coordinating veterans' Choice Program care.

However, VHA's ability to seamlessly coordinate care with community providers remains limited—even with the secure e-mail system and the

Community Viewer—because these tools only facilitate a one-way transfer of the information needed to coordinate the care veterans receive at VHA medical facilities and in the community. For the purposes of care coordination, it is important that information sharing among all participants concerned with a veteran's Choice Program or other VA community care— including VHA clinicians, the TPAs, community providers, and the veteran—is as seamless as possible. According to the federal internal control standard for information and communication, agencies should internally and externally communicate the necessary information to achieve their objectives.[63] While the secure e-mail system and Community Viewer tool provide an interim solution for VAMCs to transfer information from veterans' VA electronic health records to the TPAs and community providers, they do not provide a means by which VAMCs or veterans can (1) view step-by-step progress in scheduling appointments, or (2) electronically receive the clinical results of Choice Program or other VA community care encounters. Building such a capability into the future consolidated community care program that VA plans to implement would allow VHA to improve the care coordination processes that exist in the Choice Program.

- **Pilot programs for VAMC staff to schedule Choice Program appointments.** In July 2016 and October 2016, VHA began implementing pilot projects, whereby staff at two VAMCs took over from the TPAs the responsibility of scheduling veterans' Choice Program appointments. Specifically, VA modified its contracts with TriWest and Health Net to implement the two VAMC scheduling pilots at the Alaska VA Health Care System and the Fargo VA Health Care System, respectively. In these two locations, VAMC staff schedule veterans' appointments and send relevant clinical documentation to the Choice Program providers.[64] According to VHA officials, this had the potential

---

[63] GAO-14-704G.

[64] As part of the pilot process, the TPAs send authorizations to community providers after receiving notification that the VAMCs have scheduled appointments and before appointments occur.

to improve veterans' access to care by improving the efficiency of the Choice Program appointment scheduling process.

The results of these two VAMC scheduling pilots are particularly relevant, given that VA's RFP, as amended, for its planned consolidated community care program indicates that VAMCs—rather than TPAs—will carry out community care appointment scheduling, unless VA exercises a contract option for the TPAs to provide such services for VAMCs that request them.[65] However, while VHA officials told us that while they have taken some steps to begin evaluating the effectiveness of the pilots in improving appointment scheduling, these efforts have not been completed. The lack of an evaluation of the two VAMC scheduling pilots is inconsistent with the federal internal control standard for risk assessment, which stipulates that an agency should identify, analyze, and respond to risks related to achieving defined objectives. In addition, the federal internal control standard for monitoring calls for ongoing monitoring to assess the effectiveness of management strategies, make needed corrections if shortcomings are identified, and determine if corrective actions are achieving desired outcomes.[66] Without evaluating the results of the scheduling pilots at the Alaska and Fargo VA Health Care Systems, VA lacks assurance that VAMC staff have the potential to schedule veterans' community care appointments in a more timely manner than TPA staff otherwise would schedule them. Furthermore, VA is missing an opportunity to inform its planning and decisions for scheduling under its planned consolidated community care program.

---

[65] A May 26, 2017 amendment to VA's December 2016 RFP gave VA the option of contracting with the TPAs to carry out the appointment scheduling process for VAMCs that request these services.

[66] GAO-14-704G.

Inadequate Staffing and Ad Hoc Communication Contributed to Choice Program Access Delays, and Actions Taken Have Been Focused on the Staffing Concerns

TPA officials and managers and staff from the six selected VAMCs frequently discussed staffing- and communication-related factors that adversely affected the timeliness of veterans' Choice Program care. During the course of our review, they cited the following factors that delayed VAMCs' processing of veterans' referrals and TPAs' scheduling of appointments:

- **Staff vacancies and turnover.** TPA officials and managers and staff at selected VAMCs said that VAMCs and TPAs were initially understaffed as Choice Program implementation began.
  - *VAMCs.* Managers at the six selected VAMCs told us that after implementing the Choice Program, they hired additional community care staff, with one of them increasing its community care staffing level almost five-fold by July 2016. Some VAMC managers told us in 2016 and again in 2017 that they still struggled with staff retention and vacancies—among both managers and staff. Five of the VAMCs said they relied on overtime for their existing staff to keep up with the Choice Program workload. According to community care managers from four of the selected VAMCs, it takes about 6 months to recruit, hire, and train new community care staff, and this process could take more time if the VAMC's human resources office is also understaffed, which was the case for at least one of the six VAMCs.[67] That VAMC had not had a permanent community care manager for more than 2 years as of July

[67] In 2016, we issued a report on VHA's human capital challenges. Among other things, we found that VAMCs' human resources capacity is limited, which has affected their ability to recruit and retain VAMC staff who help deliver important services to veterans (such as staff who process referrals for VA community care). See GAO, *Veterans Health Administration: Management Attention is Needed to Address Systemic, Long-standing Human Capital Challenges,* GAO-17-30 (Washington, D.C.: Dec. 23, 2016).

2017—which covered the majority of the Choice Program's original 3-year implementation.[68]

- *TPAs*. Officials from both TPAs also told us that they initially underestimated the workload associated with scheduling Choice Program appointments, and they brought on additional staff, including sub-contractors, to better manage their workloads as utilization of the program increased. One TPA opened eight operations centers in addition to the two it already had when the Choice Program was initially implemented.[69]

- **Ineffective mechanisms for VAMCs to resolve problems.** VAMC managers and staff we interviewed also said they lacked useful mechanisms and points-of-contact when they needed to resolve issues and problems they were having with referral and appointment scheduling processes. VHA established a web-based Choice Program "issue tracker" system for VAMCs to report problems to VHA's Office of Community Care. However, staff at four of the selected VAMCs told us they rarely used the tracker and some had stopped using the tracker altogether because it took too long for VHA's Office of Community Care or the TPAs to respond and resolve the issues (if they responded at all), and they did not see the value in taking the time to report them via this mechanism. Managers at one of the VAMCs also told us about a phone line that their TPA had established to escalate and resolve urgent issues, but the TPA told the VAMC only to use it for emergencies.

- **VHA's untimely communication of Choice Program policy and process changes.** According to managers and staff at the six selected VAMCs, VA and VHA have issued numerous contract modifications and policy changes with little advanced notice throughout the Choice Program's implementation. According to

---

[68] This VAMC's leadership temporarily detailed two different managers from other areas of the VAMC to serve in the role of community care manager.

[69] Operations centers are where TPA employees who are responsible for opting veterans in to the Choice Program, scheduling veterans' appointments, and answering customer service calls from veterans and community providers work.

these VAMC managers and staff, the untimely communication of changes created confusion at the VAMC level that affected veterans' access to Choice Program care. We reviewed documentation showing that from October 2014 (when it modified the TPAs' contracts to add responsibilities related to Choice Program administration) until July 2017, VA modified each TPA's contract about 40 times. Many of these contract modifications— along with other legislative and regulatory changes that VA implemented during this period—changed VAMC or TPA processes related to Choice Program referrals and appointment scheduling. Many of the VAMC managers and staff we interviewed said they struggled to keep up with the contract modifications and policy changes, that VHA's Office of Community Care did not always leave adequate time to prepare for them, and they felt they were never really able to become proficient at new processes before additional changes occurred. This meant that training sometimes happened after the contract modifications or VHA policy changes had already gone into effect. For example, managers and staff at three of the selected VAMCs told us that they were not informed in advance about a June 2016 contract modification that required the TPAs to return Choice Program authorizations to VAMCs if they failed to schedule appointments within required time frames.[70] This contract modification had the potential to significantly increase VAMCs' workloads, because they would have to arrange veterans' care through other means once the authorizations were returned. According to individuals at two of these three VAMCs, they first heard about this change from TPA staff, rather than from VHA.

---

[70] In June 2016, VA modified its contracts with the TPAs to require the TPAs to return Choice Program authorizations when the TPAs do not meet contractual standards related to the timeliness with which they (1) review and accept referrals and (2) schedule appointments after veterans have opted into the program. Previously, the TPAs only had to return referrals if veterans had not opted in 10 days after the TPA sent a letter; there was no requirement for the TPAs to accept referrals within a certain time frame or to return authorizations if the TPAs had not scheduled appointments within required time frames after veterans opted in.

VHA took the following two actions intended to help address staffing-related factors that adversely affected the timeliness of veterans' Choice Program care.

- **Staffing tool for VAMCs to estimate needs.** In the spring of 2017, VHA developed a tool that is intended to help VAMCs project their staffing needs for the consolidated community care program VA plans to implement. VHA used workload data and site visit observations to develop the tool. Among the six selected VAMC managers we interviewed, impressions about the reasonableness of the staffing estimates generated by the community care staffing tool were mixed. For example, managers at two of the VAMCs said that the tool likely underestimated the number of staff they would need to handle referrals and appointment scheduling once VA transitions to the consolidated community care program. In contrast, managers from two other VAMCs thought that the tool's staffing estimates seemed about right.[71]

- **Co-locating TPA staff at selected VAMCs to assist with resolution of problems.** To help facilitate problem resolution between VAMCs and the TPAs as they work to schedule veterans' Choice Program appointments, VA modified the TPAs' contracts in November 2015 to allow for TPA staff to be co-located at selected VAMCs. VHA officials expected that one potential benefit of co-locating TPA staff would be that fewer veterans' Choice Program referrals would be returned to VAMCs because of missing clinical information because TPA staff could help resolve such problems locally before the TPA returned referrals. As of May 2017, TPA staff were working at 70 of VHA's 170 VAMCs—or about 40 percent of all VAMCs. Similar care coordination arrangements may exist under the consolidated community care program VA is planning to implement, if VA exercises a contract option for the TPAs to provide such services at VAMCs that request them.

---

[71] The other two VAMCs did not comment on the reasonableness of the staffing estimates generated by the staffing tool.

However, the communication-related factors that VHA and TPA officials identified as affecting the timeliness of veterans' Choice Program care remain. VHA relied on ad hoc communications such as memoranda, fact sheets, e-mails, national conference calls, and occasional web-based trainings to communicate policy and process changes to VAMCs throughout the Choice Program's implementation. Our interviews with VAMC managers and staff suggest that these were not the most effective methods of communication because messages about key changes sometimes lacked sufficient detail or failed to reach the VAMC staff responsible for implementing them in a timely manner. According to the federal internal control standard for control activities, agencies should implement control activities through their policies and procedures, which document the responsibilities of managers and staff who are responsible for implementing a program.[72] Among other things, this may include management reviewing and updating policies and day-to-day procedures in a timely manner after a significant change in the program has occurred. VHA has no comprehensive policy directive or operations manual for the Choice Program, and its broader policy directive for VA community care programs has not been updated since January 2013.[73] As a result, VAMC staff have operated in an environment that is frequently changing with no definitive reference source or sources of up-to-date policy and processes to consult, such as a comprehensive policy directive or operations manual. Instead, VAMC staff have had to keep track of the Choice Program's policy and process changes through VHA's various ad hoc communications. This poses a risk to VHA, as it increases the likelihood that VAMCs will implement new policies and processes inconsistently. In addition, there is risk that VAMC managers and

---

[72] GAO-14-704G.

[73] In October 2016 (nearly 2 years after the Choice Program was implemented), VHA issued a policy directive for the Choice Program, but it was not comprehensive because it lacked certain information that those responsible for administering the program would need to know. For example, it did not specify any time frames within which VAMC staff must complete key steps of the Choice Program referral process, such as the number of days after receiving a consult within which the VAMC's community care staff must confirm that the veteran is eligible for the Choice Program and to begin contacting the veteran to offer a referral to the program. See Veterans Health Administration, *Veterans Choice Program*, VHA Directive 1700 (Oct. 25, 2016).

staff will not always be aware of the most current policies and processes. Unless a comprehensive policy directive or operations manual is created, those risks could remain for the consolidated community care program VA is planning to establish.

Inadequate Provider Networks Affected Timely Access, but VHA Plans to Improve Available Information Related to Provider Capacity and Veteran Demand for Future TPAs

According to VAMC managers and TPA officials we interviewed, the TPAs' inadequate networks of community providers affected both the timeliness with which veterans received Choice Program care and the extent to which veterans were able to access community providers located close to their homes. In September 2015, about 11 months after the Choice Program was implemented, VA contracting officials sent corrective action letters to both TPAs, citing network adequacy (i.e., the number, mix and geographic distribution of network providers) as a concern. TPA officials we interviewed acknowledged that their networks initially were not adequate to meet demand for Choice Program care. From the TPAs' perspective, the brief transition period before the Choice Program began operations in November 2014 was not enough time to strengthen the community provider networks they had previously established under PC3, another VHA community care program. Furthermore, the TPAs told us that VA had not provided them with sufficient data on the expected demand for Choice Program care—by clinical specialty and zip code—prior to or after the Choice Program's implementation.

The overall number of community providers participating in the TPAs' Choice Program networks nationwide grew dramatically over the following year—from almost 39,000 providers in September 2015 to more than 161,000 providers as of September 2016. However, at the time of our review, managers at five of the six selected VAMCs told us that they still observed TPA network inadequacies that impeded veterans' access to Choice Program care. Similarly, managers at three VAMCs in our sample said that key community providers—including large academic medical centers—have refused to join the TPAs' networks or dropped out of the networks after joining them, often because the TPAs had not paid them in a timely manner for the services they provided.

Establishing adequate networks of Choice Program providers in rural areas has been particularly difficult. Officials at two of the three of the rural VAMCs in our sample pointed to general health care workforce shortages in rural areas as one cause for the TPAs' network inadequacy—a challenge that is not limited to the Choice Program or VA's health care system. According to a December 2015 analysis by VHA researchers, the majority of network providers in two of the three VISNs examined were located within 40 miles of VAMCs, leaving large geographic areas of these VISNs (particularly rural areas) outside the 40- mile radius with few network providers.[74] For example, only 3.8 percent of primary care providers and 3.2 percent of behavioral health providers in VISN 20 (which covers Alaska, Idaho, Oregon, and Washington) were located more than 40 miles from VAMCs within that VISN. While the areas lacking network providers generally have fewer veterans relative to other areas within these VISNs, the analysis by VHA researchers suggests that veterans living in these areas are likely to have difficulty accessing Choice Program network providers that are located closer to their homes than the nearest VAMC, which is over 40 miles away.

VA and VHA have tried to address network inadequacy that existed under the Choice Program and either have taken or plan to take additional actions to address this issue for the community care program VA plans to implement, including the following.

- **Establishment of Choice Program provider agreement process.** To help address inadequacies in the TPAs' provider networks and improve veterans' access to care under the Choice Program, VHA

---

[74] Evan Carey, Paula Langner, and Michael Ho, *VACA Spatial Evaluation: Quantitative Results,* a report prepared for the Department of Veterans Affairs, Veterans Health Administration, Dec. 28, 2015. The analysis examined the distribution of network providers participating in the Choice Program in VISN 10, which covers Ohio, Indiana, and Michigan; VISN 19, which covers Colorado, Montana, Oklahoma, Utah, and Wyoming; and VISN 20, which covers Alaska, Idaho, Oregon, and Washington.

established the Choice Program provider agreement process in February 2016. This process allowed VAMCs to establish agreements with community providers, schedule veterans' appointments, and reimburse the providers directly (using Choice Program funds) when the TPAs failed to schedule veterans' appointments for reasons relating to network inadequacy, among others.[75] Originally, the VAMCs were required to send veterans' referrals to the TPAs and wait for them to be returned before they could proceed with arranging care through a Choice Program provider agreement. While this process had the potential to increase the availability of providers for the Choice Program, it did not immediately improve the timeliness of veterans' Choice Program care because veterans still had to wait for as long as it took the VAMCs to send their referrals to the TPAs and for TPAs to return them before the VAMCs could proceed with arranging care through Choice Program provider agreements. According to the policies and contractual requirements that were in effect at the time, it could have taken up to 40 calendar days after a VHA clinician first identified the veteran's need for care until the TPA returned the referral and the VAMC could proceed with arranging care through a Choice Program provider agreement. However, in March 2017, VHA updated the Choice Program provider agreement process so that— if the TPAs were returning a high volume of a VAMC's referrals for one or more types of care—the VAMC could seek approval from its VISN and VHA's Office of Community Care to bypass the TPA and proceed directly to arranging that type of care through Choice

---

[75] Specifically, VAMCs could proceed with arranging care through the Choice Program provider agreement process if the TPAs returned veterans' referrals for any of these reasons, among others: (1) the TPA had no network provider available for the service VA requested; (2) the veteran requested a specific community provider that was not part of the TPA's network; (3) the TPA failed to complete the steps of the appointment scheduling process within the time frames that were outlined in its contract; (4) the TPA was unable to reach the veteran via telephone or letter when attempting to schedule the appointment; and (5) the TPA did not schedule the appointment on a day and time that was convenient for the veteran. In addition, VAMCs were permitted to arrange care through the Choice Program provider agreement process (and pay for it using Choice Program funds) when the veteran needed services that were not covered under the TPAs' contracts, such as dental and home health services.

Program provider agreements. This had the potential to improve the timeliness of veterans' access to Choice Program care because it eliminated the steps of sending referrals to the TPAs and waiting for them to be returned.

- **Improving quality of information given to future TPAs.** To help inform the recruitment of network providers for the consolidated community care program VA plans to establish, VA plans to provide future TPAs more robust data than they provided the current TPAs at the start of the Choice Program. In particular, VA's RFP for the consolidated community care program, as amended, indicates that VA will provide (1) zip-code-level data on the number of authorizations that were issued in fiscal year 2015 for specific types of care (e.g., chemotherapy and obstetrics) and (2) VAMC-level data on the clinical specialties with the greatest wait times for appointments at VAMCs. These local-level data could help TPAs estimate the number of network providers of various specialties they will need to recruit in specific localities if awarded a contract for the consolidated community care program that VA is planning to implement.

- **Performing market assessments.** In preparation for the consolidated community care program VA plans to establish, VA and VHA officials are planning to conduct market assessments in 96 markets nationwide. Through these market assessments, officials told us, VA will (1) examine the clinical capacity that currently exists within VHA medical facilities and among community providers, (2) assess veterans' current and future demand for health care services, and (3) develop long-term plans for ensuring that veterans will have access to high-quality health care services— whether they receive care from VHA clinicians or from community providers. According to VHA officials, the market assessments will help inform network provider recruitment efforts for the consolidated community care program VA is planning to implement. In addition, VHA officials told us that the market assessments will help VISN- and VAMC-level leaders make more informed, strategic decisions about whether it is more efficient to maintain or build capacity for delivering particular types of care within VHA medical facilities, or if they should routinely purchase certain types of care in the community. In November 2017, VHA officials told us that they expect to begin conducting the market assessments early in calendar year 2018, and the officials estimate that it will take about 18 months to complete assessments for all 96 markets.

CONCLUSION

The Choice Program is approaching the end of its life, and with plans to consolidate it with VA's other community care programs, opportunities to improve the program are diminishing. Congress created the Choice Program in 2014 in response to longstanding challenges in veterans' access to care delivered within VHA medical facilities. However, we found numerous operational and oversight weaknesses with VHA's management of scheduling veterans' medical appointments through the Choice Program. While it may not be feasible for VA and VHA to implement corrective actions to address all of our findings before the Choice Program ends, it is imperative that VA incorporate lessons learned from the Choice Program when it implements the consolidated community care program it has planned.

First, we found VHA's process for scheduling appointments for veterans through the Choice Program was not consistent with statutory requirements. The Choice Act requires veterans to receive care no more than 30 days from the date an appointment is deemed clinically appropriate or from the date the veteran prefers to receive care; however, we found that veterans could potentially wait up to 70 calendar days to receive routine care through the Choice Program. In effect, we found that in 2016, some veterans' actual wait times far exceeded 30 days. Although VA has made some relevant contract modifications and issued guidance to address Choice Program wait times, VHA has not adjusted the Choice Program's appointment scheduling process or established timeliness standards for all steps of the process. In addition, VHA's monitoring of access to Choice Program care has been limited by incomplete and unreliable data. In particular, the data VHA uses preclude it from accurately identifying the number of days that occur within each phase of the process, from initial referral to the actual appointment. Furthermore, a lack of controls has allowed for inappropriate changes to be made in veterans' clinically indicated dates and routine versus urgent care categorizations, affecting VA's ability to monitor whether veterans are receiving Choice Program care in a timely manner. The lack of reliable data and performance measures also hinders VHA's ability to oversee the program and identify problems and corrective actions. Further, we found that VHA is missing out on opportunities to enhance its design of the planned consolidated community care program. For example, VHA has not fully evaluated its pilot programs for scheduling appointments nor developed tools such as a mechanism that would allow the seamless sharing of information between VHA and the TPAs. Lastly, we found that VHA often relied on inefficient, ad hoc methods of sharing information (such as memoranda, fact sheets and emails), which often failed to reach the VAMC managers and staff responsible for implementing the program.

After the Choice Program ends, VA anticipates that veterans will continue to receive care from non-VHA providers under the consolidated community care program that it is planning to implement. VA's and VHA's design of the future program can benefit from the lessons learned under the Choice Program. Ignoring these lessons learned and the challenges that have arisen under the Choice Program as VA and VHA design the future consolidated program would only increase VA's risk for not being able to ensure that all veterans will receive timely access to care in the community.

RECOMMENDATIONS FOR EXECUTIVE ACTION

To ensure that VA and VHA incorporate lessons learned from the Choice Program as they develop and implement a consolidated VA community care program, we are making the following 10 recommendations:

- The Under Secretary for Health should establish an achievable wait-time goal for the consolidated community care program that VA plans to implement that will permit VHA to monitor whether veterans are receiving VA community care within time frames that are comparable to the amount of time they would otherwise wait to receive care at VHA medical facilities. (Recommendation 1)
- The Under Secretary for Health should design an appointment scheduling process for the consolidated community care program that VA plans to implement that sets forth time frames within which (1) veterans' referrals must be processed, (2) veterans' appointments must be scheduled, and (3) veterans' appointments must occur, which are consistent with the wait-time goal VHA has established for the program. (Recommendation 2)
- The Under Secretary for Health should establish a mechanism that will allow VHA to systematically monitor the average number of days it takes for VAMCs to prepare referrals, for VAMCs or TPAs to schedule veterans' appointments, and for veterans' appointments to occur, under the consolidated community care program that VA plans to implement. (Recommendation 3)
- The Under Secretary for Health should implement a mechanism to prevent veterans' clinically indicated dates from being modified by individuals other than VHA clinicians when veterans are referred to the consolidated community care program that VA plans to implement. (Recommendation 4)

- The Under Secretary for Health should implement a mechanism to separate clinically urgent referrals and authorizations from those for which the VAMC or the TPA has decided to expedite appointment scheduling for administrative reasons. (Recommendation 5)
- The Under Secretary for Health should (1) establish oversight mechanisms to ensure that VHA is collecting reliable data on the reasons that VAMC or TPA staff are unsuccessful in scheduling veterans' appointments through the consolidated community care program VA plans to implement, and (2) demonstrate that it has corrected any identified deficiencies. (Recommendation 6)
- The Secretary of Veterans Affairs should ensure that the contracts for the consolidated community care program VA plans to implement include performance metrics that will allow VHA to monitor average driving times between veterans' homes and the practice locations of community providers that participate in the TPAs' networks. (Recommendation 7)
- The Secretary of Veterans Affairs should establish a system for the consolidated community care program VA plans to implement to help facilitate seamless, efficient information sharing among VAMCs, VHA clinicians, TPAs, community providers, and veterans. Specifically, this system should allow all of these entities to electronically exchange information for the purposes of care coordination. (Recommendation 8)
- The Under Secretary for Health should conduct a comprehensive evaluation of the outcomes of the two appointment scheduling pilots it established at the Alaska and Fargo VA Health Care Systems (where VAMC staff, rather than TPA staff, are responsible for scheduling veterans' Choice Program appointments), which should include a comparison of the timeliness with which VAMC staff and TPA staff completed each step of the Choice Program appointment scheduling process, as well as the overall timeliness with which veterans received appointments. (Recommendation 9)

- The Under Secretary for Health should issue a comprehensive policy directive and operations manual for the consolidated community care program VA plans to implement and ensure that these documents are reviewed and updated in a timely manner after any significant changes to the program occur. (Recommendation 10)

AGENCY COMMENTS AND OUR EVALUATION

VA provided written comments on a draft of this chapter, which are reprinted in Appendix VII. In its comments, VA concurred with 8 of our 10 recommendations and described its plans for implementing them. VA stated that VHA's Office of Community Care will work collaboratively with other VA and VHA offices to evaluate modifications to the current wait-time goals and measurement processes so that wait times for VA community care can be compared to wait times for care delivered at VHA medical facilities.

VA did not concur with our recommendation to implement a mechanism to separate clinically urgent referrals and authorizations from those that are designated as urgent for administrative reasons. VA stated that because VAMC staff (rather than TPA staff) will be responsible for scheduling veterans' appointments under the consolidated community care program it plans to implement, there would no longer be a need to separate clinically urgent referrals from those that need to be administratively expedited. However, we maintain that our recommendation is warranted. In particular, we found that VA's data did not always accurately reflect the timeliness of urgent care because both VAMC and TPA staff inappropriately re-categorized some routine care referrals and authorizations as urgent ones for reasons unrelated to the veterans' health conditions. Regardless of whether VAMC staff or TPA staff are responsible for appointment scheduling, VA will need to ensure that it uses reliable data to monitor the extent to which veterans receive urgent care within required time frames. Without a means of separating clinically urgent referrals and authorizations from ones for which the scheduling process must be administratively expedited, VA's data on the timeliness of urgent care will continue to be unreliable.

VA agreed in principle with our recommendation to issue a comprehensive policy directive and operations manual, but stated in its comments that it would wait to determine whether a comprehensive policy directive is needed until after the consolidated community care program has been fully implemented and any interim implementation challenges have been resolved. However, when implementing a new program, it is important that agencies establish the program's structure, responsibilities, and authorities at the beginning to help ensure that the new program's objectives are met. Relying on outdated policies and unreliable communication methods increases VA's risk of encountering foreseeable challenges. Without issuing a comprehensive policy directive and operations manual before the start of the new program, VA risks experiencing untimely communication issues similar to those that affected veterans' access to care throughout the Choice Program's implementation. A comprehensive policy directive and operations manual that could be updated as changes occur would give VAMCs a definitive source of real-time, up-to-date information and reduce the likelihood that VAMCs will implement new policies and processes inconsistently under the future program.

We are sending copies of this chapter to the Secretary of Veterans Affairs, the Under Secretary for Health, appropriate congressional committees, and other interested parties. This chapter is also available at no charge on the GAO Web site at http://www.gao.gov.

Sharon M. Silas
Acting Director, Health Care

A. Nicole Clowers
Managing Director, Health Care

LIST OF ADDRESSEES

The Honorable Johnny Isakson
Chairman

The Honorable Jon Tester
Ranking Member
Committee on Veterans' Affairs
United States Senate

The Honorable John Boozman
Chairman

The Honorable Brian Schatz
Ranking Member
Subcommittee on Military Construction,
Veterans Affairs, and Related Agencies
Committee on Appropriations
United States Senate

The Honorable Phil Roe
Chairman

The Honorable Tim Walz
Ranking Member
Committee on Veterans' Affairs
House of Representatives

The Honorable John Carter
Chairman

The Honorable Debbie Wasserman Schultz
Ranking Member

Subcommittee on Military Construction,
Veterans Affairs, and Related Agencies
Committee on Appropriations
House of Representatives

The Honorable Richard Blumenthal
United States Senate

The Honorable Mike Enzi
United States Senate

The Honorable John McCain
United States Senate

The Honorable Evan Jenkins
House of Representatives

APPENDIX I: SCOPE AND METHODOLOGY FOR EXAMINING CHOICE PROGRAM WAIT TIMES AND THE DATA VHA USES TO MONITOR ACCESS

To examine selected veterans' actual wait times to receive routine care and urgent care through the Choice Program and the information VHA uses to monitor access to care under the program, we took five key steps. We (1) analyzed Choice Program appointment wait times for selected veterans using a sample of 196 Choice Program authorizations for routine and urgent care; (2) reviewed VHA's analysis of Choice Program appointment wait times for a sample of about 5,000 Choice Program authorizations; (3) reviewed data VHA uses to monitor the timeliness of Choice Program care and reasons that the TPAs have returned Choice Program referrals without making appointments; (4) interviewed VA, VHA, and TPA officials; and (5) reviewed federal internal control standards, as follows.

1) **Our analysis of Choice Program wait times for a sample of 196 authorizations.** To analyze the timeliness of Choice Program appointment scheduling and completion for a sample of veterans, we selected six VAMCs and a random, non-generalizable sample of 196 authorizations for veterans who were referred to the Choice Program by those six VAMCs between January 2016 and April 2016.[76] We judgmentally selected the six VAMCs to include variation in geographic location, with three VAMCs that serve rural veteran populations and three VAMCs that serve urban veteran populations. In addition, three of the VAMCs were served by Health Net, and three were served by TriWest. (See Table 5.)

To select our random, non-generalizable sample of 196 Choice Program authorizations, we obtained VA data on all authorizations created by the TPAs between January and April 2016 for veterans who were referred to the program by the six VAMCs we selected—a universe of about 55,000 authorizations. From these 55,000 authorizations, we randomly selected:

- 55 routine care authorizations (about 10 authorizations per VAMC) for which the TPAs scheduled appointments for veterans,
- 53 urgent care authorizations (about 10 authorizations per VAMC) for which the TPAs scheduled appointments for veterans, and
- 88 routine and urgent care authorizations (about 15 authorizations per VAMC) that the TPAs returned to VA without scheduling appointments for any one of the following three reasons—(1) VA requested the authorization be returned, (2) VA data were missing from the referral, and (3) the veteran declined or did not want Choice Program care.[77]

---

[76] These were the most recent Choice Program authorization data that were available when we began our review. We did not assess whether these authorizations met the Choice Act's eligibility requirements. We selected our sample and conducted our analysis based on contract requirements that were in effect as of April 2016. Certain contract requirements were later modified.

[77] We limited our sample of returned authorizations to these three return reasons because we wanted to determine if the return reasons entered by the TPAs could be substantiated by evidence from the veterans' VA electronic health records.

Table 5. Department of Veterans Affairs (VA) Medical Centers (VAMC) GAO Selected for Its Review of the Veterans Choice Program (Choice Program)

n/a	n/a	Choice Program third party administrator that serves the VAMC	
VAMC (location)	Rural or urban[a]	Health Net Federal Services	TriWest Healthcare Alliance
Togus VAMC (Augusta, ME)	rural	yes	n/a
Muskogee VAMC (Muskogee, OK)	rural	n/a	yes
Alaska VA Health Care System (Anchorage, AK)	urban – location rural – population served	n/a	yes
VA Eastern Colorado Health Care System (Denver, CO)	urban	yes	n/a
VA Northern California Health Care System (Mather, CA)	urban	n/a	yes
Durham VAMC (Durham, NC)	urban	yes	n/a

Source: GAO | GAO-18-281.

[a]In this table, urban and rural classifications are based on U.S. Census measures of the population density where the VAMC is located, unless otherwise noted.

For all 196 Choice Program authorizations in our sample, we manually reviewed VHA documentation (specifically, the veterans' VA electronic health records) and TPA documentation to track the number of calendar days that elapsed at each step of the Choice Program appointment scheduling process.[78] For the authorizations that the TPAs returned to the VAMCs without making appointments, we examined VHA and TPA documentation to determine whether the veterans eventually obtained care through other means—such as through another VA community care program, a different

---

[78] In this report, "days" refers to calendar days, unless otherwise indicated.

Choice Program referral, or at a VHA medical facility—and how long it took to receive that care. Determining whether veterans in our sample experienced clinical harm or adverse clinical outcomes because of delays in the VAMCs' or TPAs' processing of their referrals and authorizations was outside the scope of our review.

We selected our sample of 55 routine care and 53 urgent care authorizations for which the TPAs succeeded in scheduling appointments to include only authorizations for which the TPAs did not meet VA's appointment scheduling goals at one phase of the appointment scheduling process: when the TPAs attempt to schedule appointments after the veterans have opted in to the program.[79] This was to ensure that our sample included only authorizations for which scheduling was delayed, so that we could examine the potential causes of appointment scheduling delays and whether delays also occurred at other phases of the process (such as when VAMCs were preparing the veterans' referrals or when the TPAs were attempting to reach the veterans for them to opt in to the program).[80] We omitted this phase of the appointment scheduling process when calculating the timeliness of appointment completion for the 55 routine care authorizations and 53 urgent care authorizations in our sample. Rather than reporting veterans' overall wait times for these authorizations, we report the average number of calendar days that elapsed (1) while VAMCs were preparing veterans' Choice Program referrals, (2) while the TPAs were attempting to reach veterans for them to opt in to the program, and (3) while veterans waited to attend their appointments after the TPAs succeeded in scheduling them. To assess the reliability of the authorization data we used, we interviewed

---

[79] Under VA's contracts with the TPAs, VA requires that the TPAs schedule routine Choice Program appointments within 5 business days after veterans opt into the Choice Program. VA also requires that the TPAs schedule veterans' urgent Choice Program appointments and provide care within 2 business days after veterans opt in to the Choice Program.

[80] As we discuss in this report, VHA could not provide complete, reliable data that would have allowed us to include authorizations in our sample that were delayed at other points of the Choice Program appointment scheduling process, such as the period when VAMCs prepare referrals for the TPAs or the period between the TPAs' receipt of referrals and initiation of appointment scheduling.

knowledgeable agency officials, manually reviewed the content of the data, and electronically tested it for missing values. We concluded that these data were sufficiently reliable for the purposes of our reporting objectives. The findings from our review of Choice Program authorizations cannot be generalized beyond the VAMCs and the veterans' Choice Program authorizations we reviewed.

2) **VHA's analysis of Choice Program wait times for a sample of about 5,000 authorizations.** We obtained from VHA's Office of Community Care the results of a nationwide analysis of Choice Program appointment timeliness it conducted in February 2017. Specifically, VHA directed its VAMCs to manually review veterans' health records and TPA documentation and report observations for a non-generalizable sample of about 5,000 randomly selected Choice Program authorizations that were created between July and September of 2016.[81] The sample was limited to authorizations for Choice Program appointments that had been scheduled for time-eligible veterans who needed four types of specialty care— mammography, gastroenterology, cardiology, and neurology. According to VHA officials, they limited their analysis to these four types of care because delayed treatment for any of these specialties could cause adverse health outcomes for patients. To assess the reliability of VHA's data, we manually reviewed the results of its analysis and interviewed knowledgeable agency officials about potential outliers. We concluded that VHA's data were sufficiently reliable for the purposes of our reporting objective. The results of VHA's analysis cannot be generalized beyond the sample of Choice Program authorizations that it reviewed.

---

[81] The VAMCs were directed to report to VHA the dates on which key steps of the Choice Program appointment scheduling process occurred for each authorization—such as the date the veteran's need for care was identified, the date the VAMC sent the veteran's Choice Program referral to the TPA, the date the TPA succeeded in scheduling an appointment, and the date on which the scheduled appointment was to occur.

3) **VHA data on timeliness of Choice Program appointments and the reasons TPAs return referrals without making appointments.** To evaluate the information VHA uses to monitor access to care under the Choice Program, we reviewed data that VHA collects to monitor the timeliness with which the TPAs schedule appointments and the timeliness with which appointments occur after the TPAs have scheduled them. We also reviewed and tested the reliability of VHA data on the reasons the TPAs have returned Choice Program referrals to VAMCs without scheduling appointments, which may offer insights about access to care (e.g., the percentage of referrals that are returned due to a lack of providers in the TPAs' networks).

4) **Interviews with officials.** We interviewed VA, VHA, and TPA officials responsible for administering the Choice Program contracts and overseeing implementation of the program. We interviewed these officials to gain an understanding of the processes they followed and the information they used to monitor veterans' access to Choice Program care.

5) **Federal internal control standards.** We examined the results of our and VHA's analyses and the information VHA uses to monitor veterans' access to care under the program in the context of federal standards for internal control for (1) information and communication and (2) monitoring.[82] The internal control standard for information and communication relates to management's ability to use quality information to achieve the entity's objectives. The internal control standard for monitoring relates to establishing activities to monitor the quality of performance over time and evaluating the results.

---

[82] GAO, *Standards for Internal Control in the Federal Government*, GAO-14-704G (Washington, D.C.: Sept. 2014).

APPENDIX II: PROCESS FOR VETERANS TO OBTAIN DEPARTMENT OF VETERANS AFFAIRS (VA) CHOICE PROGRAM CARE IF THEY ARE TIME-ELIGIBLE[A]

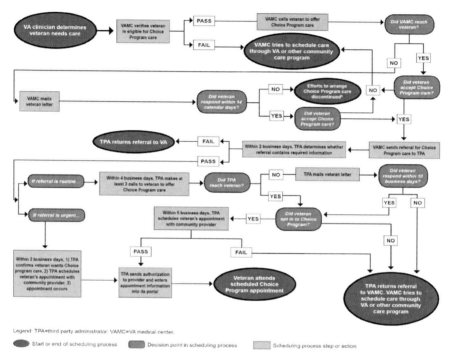

Legend: TPA=third party administrator: VAMC=VA medical center.

Source: GAO illustration based on VHA information. | GAO-18-281.

[a]VHA uses the time-eligible appointment scheduling process when the services needed are not available at a VHA medical facility or are not available within allowable wait times.

[b]If the veteran does not respond to the letter within 14 calendar days, a notification is sent to the veteran's VA clinician so that they can determine if additional action should be taken.

Figure 5. Process for Veterans to Obtain Department of Veterans Affairs (VA) Choice Program Care if They Are Time-Eligible.[a]

APPENDIX III: PROCESS FOR VETERANS TO OBTAIN DEPARTMENT OF VETERANS AFFAIRS (VA) CHOICE PROGRAM CARE IF THEY ARE DISTANCE-ELIGIBLE[A]

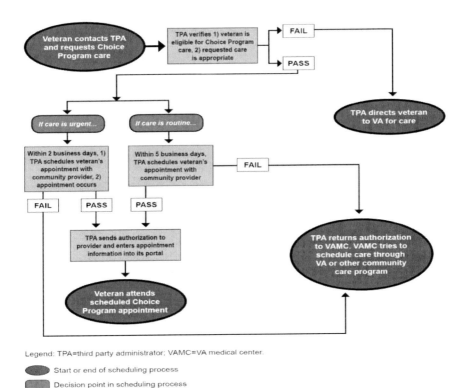

Legend: TPA=third party administrator; VAMC=VA medical center.

Start or end of scheduling process

Decision point in scheduling process

Scheduling process step or action

Source: GAO illustration based on VHA information. | GAO-18-281.

[a]VHA uses the distance-eligible appointment scheduling process when veterans reside more than 40 miles from a VHA medical facility or meet other travel-related criteria.

Figure 6. Process for Veterans to Obtain Department of Veterans Affairs (VA) Choice Program Care if They Are Distance-Eligible.[a]

APPENDIX IV: COMPARISON OF PROCESSES FOR ARRANGING CHOICE PROGRAM AND INDIVIDUALLY AUTHORIZED COMMUNITY CARE

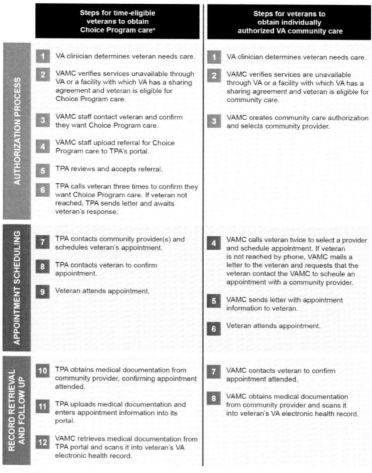

Legend: TPA=third party administrator; VAMC=VA medical center.

Source: GAO illustration on VHA information. | GAO-18-281.

aThe Veterans Health Administration (VHA) uses the time-eligible appointment scheduling process when the services needed are not available at a VHA medical facility or are not available within allowable wait times.

Figure 7. Comparison of Processes for Arranging Choice Program and Individually Authorized Department of Veterans Affairs (VA) Community Care.

APPENDIX V: PROCESS FOR OBTAINING THE CLINICAL RESULTS OF CHOICE PROGRAM APPOINTMENTS

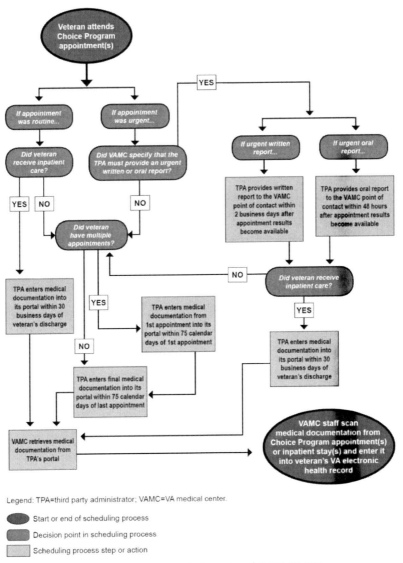

Source: GAO illustration based on VHA information. | GAO-18-281.

Figure 8. Process for the Department of Veterans Affairs (VA) to Obtain the Clinical Results of Veterans' Choice Program Appointments.

APPENDIX VI: SELECTED ACTIONS TAKEN BY VA AND VHA TO ADDRESS CHOICE PROGRAM ACCESS ISSUES

We found 21 actions that the Department of Veterans Affairs (VA) and the Veterans Health Administration (VHA) took after the Choice Program's November 2014 implementation that were intended to help address issues related to veterans' access to care. Table 6, below, provides a chronological summary of the actions VA and VHA had taken as of August 2017 and the issues they were intended to address.

Table 6. Selected Actions Taken by the Department of Veterans Affairs (VA) and the Veterans Health Administration (VHA) between November 2014 and August 2017 to Address Choice Program Access Issues

Action taken (implementation time frame)	Description of action	Issue(s) that action was intended to help address
1. Updated Choice Program eligibility criteria for distance-eligible veterans (Apr. 2015)	VA published an interim final rule that changed how it determined whether veterans were distance-eligible for the Choice Program.[a] Originally, VA used straight-line or geodesic distance to determine whether veterans resided more than 40 miles from a VHA medical facility. However, VA later changed this standard so that eligibility determinations would instead be made on the basis of driving distance, which helped simplify Choice Program administrative processes.	administrative burden
2. Established an outbound call process (Sept. –Nov. 2015)	VA modified the third party administrators' (TPA) contracts to establish an outbound call process. It required that the TPAs contact veterans at least three times by telephone after receiving VAMCs' referrals, to confirm the veterans want to opt in to the Choice Program and have the TPA proceed with appointment scheduling. Previously, veterans had to contact the TPAs on their own and opt in to the Choice Program after VAMCs sent their referrals to the TPAs, a confusing process that contributed to delays in veterans accessing Choice Program care.	administrative burden

Action taken (implementation time frame)	Description of action	Issue(s) that action was intended to help address
3. Updated veteran eligibility criteria (Sept. –Dec. 2015)	VA modified the TPAs' contracts and published an interim final rule, and VHA issued guidance to its VAMCs regarding the implementation of statutory updates to Choice Program eligibility criteria for veterans. Specifically, they allowed all veterans who are enrolled in the VA health care system (not just those who were enrolled at the time the Choice Act became law) to be eligible to obtain care through the Choice Program, and they implemented the "unusual or excessive travel burden" eligibility criterion.[b] These changes had the potential to simplify Choice Program administrative processes.	administrative burden
4. Created a standard Choice Program referral form (Oct. –Dec. 2015)	VHA introduced a standard form for VAMCs to use when sending veterans' Choice Program referrals to the TPAs, and VA modified the TPAs' contracts to account for use of this form. Previously, the TPAs had to wait for VA to send them electronic updates to their eligibility files, which did not always happen before the TPAs received the VAMCs' referrals. With the standardized form, VAMCs could attest to veterans' eligibility, which removed the step of the TPAs having to verify eligibility through another source.	administrative burden
5. Co-located TPA staff at selected VAMCs (Nov. 2015)	VA modified the TPAs' contracts to allow for TPA staff to be co-located at selected VAMCs—an action that VHA officials said could help improve communication between VAMC and TPA staff and potentially speed up the process of Choice Program appointment scheduling. As of May 2017, 70 of VHA's 170 VAMCs had co-located TPA staff.	staffing
6. Expanded standard episode of care from 60 days to 1 year (eff. Dec. 2015 and active Jan. 2016)	VA modified the TPAs' contracts and updated its policies to implement a Choice Act amendment that increased the time limit on Choice Program episodes of care from 60 days to 1 year.[c] According to VA and TPA officials, this had the potential to significantly reduce TPAs' and VAMCs' administrative burden associated with re-authorizing care when veterans' Choice Program authorizations expired.	administrative burden

Table 6. (Continued)

Action taken (implementation time frame)	Description of action	Issue(s) that action was intended to help address
7. Automated VAMCs' preparation of Choice Program referrals (Early 2016)	VHA established a web-based tool—called the "referral documentation" (REFDOC) tool, which automates the process by which VAMC staff compile clinical information for veterans' Choice Program referrals. VHA's initial analyses for the REFDOC tool's effectiveness found that it sped up the process of preparing Choice Program referrals by about 20 minutes per referral.	administrative burden
8. Clarified eligibility requirements for community providers of mental health services (Feb. 2016)	VA modified the TPAs' contracts to clarify that mental health providers with Masters-level degrees were eligible to participate in the TPAs' Choice Program networks, which had the potential to help address network adequacy issues.	network inadequacy
9. Established Choice Provider Agreement process (Feb. 2016 –June 2016)	VHA established a process that allowed VAMCs to use Choice Program funds to arrange community care for veterans when the TPAs could not arrange such care—either because the services were not covered under the Choice Program contracts (e.g., dental and home health services) or because the TPAs returned Choice Program authorizations to VAMCs without scheduling appointments. In part, this process was intended to address network inadequacy, which was causing the TPAs to return authorizations to VAMCs.	network inadequacy
10. De-coupled medical documentation from payment of community providers' Choice Program claims (Mar. 2016)	VA modified the TPAs' contracts by relaxing requirements related to the amount of time community providers have to return medical records associated with an episode of routine care. Previously, the TPAs were not allowed to pay community providers' Choice Program claims until the TPAs received medical records from the providers, but the contract modification removed this requirement. This action had the potential to simplify the TPAs' post-appointment follow-up processes. It was also intended to help address delays in the TPAs' payments to community providers, which had been causing some to drop out of the TPAs' networks.	administrative burden, network inadequacy

Action taken (implementation time frame)	Description of action	Issue(s) that action was intended to help address
11. Required TPAs to return referrals to VAMCs if appointments are not scheduled within required time frames (June 2016)	VA modified the TPAs' contracts to require the TPAs to return Choice Program authorizations when the TPAs did not meet contractual standards related to the timeliness with which they (1) reviewed and accepted referrals and (2) scheduled appointments after veterans opted into the program. Previously, the TPAs had to return referrals only if veterans had not opted in 10 days after the TPA sent a letter. This contract modification had the potential to limit appointment scheduling delays that would be attributable to the TPAs. It also had the potential to address network adequacy issues, which was a common reason that TPAs were unable to meet appointment scheduling timeliness requirements.	administrative burden, network inadequacy
12. Created two pilot programs for VAMC staff to schedule Choice Program appointments (July 2016 and Oct. 2016)	VA modified the TPAs' contracts to establish pilot programs at two VAMCs (specifically, the Alaska VA Health Care System and the Fargo VA Health Care System), where VAMC staff took over Choice Program appointment scheduling responsibilities from the TPAs. In these two locations, VAMC staff scheduled veterans' appointments and sent relevant clinical documentation to the Choice Program providers, and the TPAs sent authorizations to the Choice Program providers before veterans attended their appointments. This had the potential to improve the efficiency of the Choice Program appointment scheduling process in the two pilot locations.	administrative burden
13. Established a real-time, web-based communication tool for VAMCs and TPAs (Aug. 2016 –Jan. 2017)	VHA implemented a real-time communication tool (specifically, a web-based chat program), which VAMC staff could use to communicate with TPA officials about problems that arose with specific Choice Program referrals (such as missing clinical information), or patterns of problems that emerged with Choice Program referrals.	administrative burden
14. Established qualifications for certain types of non-federal and	VA modified the TPAs' contracts to revise Choice Program eligibility requirements for providers of women's health care services, audiology, pediatrics, and optometry.	network inadequacy

Table 6. (Continued)

Action taken (implementation time frame)	Description of action	Issue(s) that action was intended to help address
non-Medicare participating providers to participate in the TPAs' Choice Program networks (Jan. –Feb. 2017)	These contract modifications implemented a July 2015 statutory change, which allowed these types of providers to participate in the TPAs' Choice Program networks.[d] Previously, the Choice Act limited the TPAs' networks to providers that either (1) participated in the Medicare program or (2) were affiliated with the Department of Defense, the Indian Health Service, or federally qualified health centers.[e]	
15. Clarified requirements relating to the provision of durable medical equipment during episodes of Choice Program care (Feb. –Mar. 2017)	VA modified the TPAs' contracts to clarify requirements relating to the provision of durable medical equipment —specifically, how the TPAs are to coordinate with VAMCs to obtain durable medical equipment during episodes of routine care, and the extent to which VA will cover durable medical equipment (such as crutches, slings, and canes) supplied by community providers during episodes of urgent care. This had the potential to improve the process of delivering durable medical equipment to veterans who need it and streamline discharge processes when veterans are leaving inpatient settings of care.	administrative burden
16. Added tele-mental health services to the TPAs' contracts (Mar. –May 2017)	VA modified the TPAs' contracts to permit psychologists, psychiatrists, licensed clinical social workers, and advanced registered nurse practitioners to provide tele-mental health services through the TPAs' networks. This has the potential to improve the availability of network providers for veterans who reside in rural locations.	network inadequacy
17. Acquired a secure e-mail system for transmitting veterans' medical records (Mar. –May 2017)	VA acquired software that allows VAMC managers and staff to e-mail encrypted files containing veterans' medical records to the TPAs and Choice Program community providers. Only the intended recipient can decrypt and respond to messages containing the files. This action is intended to improve the efficiency of coordinating veterans' Choice Program care and address potential security risks associated with printing paper copies of veterans' medical records and sending them to the TPAs or community providers via fax or U.S. mail.	administrative burden

Action taken (implementation time frame)	Description of action	Issue(s) that action was intended to help address
18. Approved standard sets of clinical services that are to be authorized whenever veterans are referred to the Choice Program for certain types of care (April 2017)	VHA approved standardized episodes of care—or "bundles" of clinically necessary medical services and procedures—that are to be authorized whenever veterans are referred to community providers for specified types of care. VHA approved standardized episodes of care for 15 different types of care, including physical therapy, maternity care, and optometry, and planned to roll out additional standardized episodes of care over time. This had the potential to simplify the VAMCs' preparation of veterans' Choice Program referrals and TPAs' processing of authorizations.	administrative burden
19. Implemented a new law that made VA the primary coordinator of benefits for veterans with other health insurance (Apr. 2017)	VHA implemented an April 19, 2017, law that made VA the primary coordinator of benefits when veterans with other health insurance use the Choice Program for nonservice-connected care.[f] This had the potential to simplify VAMCs', TPAs', and community providers' administrative processes. Previously, VAMCs had to determine whether the health care services the veteran was attempting to access through the Choice Program were related to the veteran's service-connected disability. If they were not, community providers had to collect other health insurance copayments and bill veterans' other health insurance prior to seeking Choice Program payments from the TPAs. Under the new law, community providers will bill only the TPAs, and VA will later bill veterans' other health insurance for nonservice-connected care.	administrative burden
20. Provided a mechanism for community providers to have access to veterans' VA electronic health records (May 2017)	VA developed a secure, web-based application called the Community Viewer, which allows community providers to remotely view veterans' VA electronic health records. VAMC staff create usernames and passwords for approved community providers, who then have access only to assigned veterans' medical information. The Community Viewer is intended to improve the efficiency of care coordination and sharing health information between veterans' VHA clinicians and community providers.	administrative burden

Table 6. (Continued)

Action taken (implementation time frame)	Description of action	Issue(s) that action was intended to help address
21. Provided a tool for VAMCs to analyze their future staffing needs(May 2017)	VHA developed a tool that is intended to help VAMCs project their future Provided a tool for VAMCs to staffing needs. VHA used workload data and site visit observations to develop the tool.	staffing

Legend: ☎ = administrative burden

🖆 = staffing, feedback mechanisms for VAMCs, and VHA's communication of policy and process changes

📶 = network inadequacy

Source: GAO analysis of VA and VHA information. | GAO-18-281

[a]80 Fed. Reg. 22906 (2015).

[b]Pub. L. No. 114-41, § 4005(a), 129 Stat. 443, 464 (2015).

[c]Pub. L. No. 114-41, § 4005(c), 129 Stat. 443, 464 (2015).

[d]Pub. L. No. 114-41, § 4005(c), 129 Stat. 443, 464 (2015).

[e]Pub. L. No. 113-146, § 101(a)(1)(B), 128 Stat. 1754, 1756 (2014).

[f]Pub. L. No. 115-26, § 2, 131 Stat. 129 (2017).

APPENDIX VII: COMMENTS FROM THE DEPARTMENT OF VETERAN'S AFFAIRS

DEPARTMENT OF VETERANS AFFAIRS
WASHINGTON DC 20420
May16, 2018

Ms. A. Nicole Clowers
Managing Director
Health Care
U.S. Government Accountability Office

Dear Ms. Clowers:

The Department of Veterans Affairs (VA) has reviewed the Government Accountability Office's (GAO) draft report, *"VETERANS CHOICE*

PROGRAM: Improvements Needed to Address Access-Related Challenges as VA Plans · Consolidation of its Community Care Programs" (GA0-18-281).

The enclosure provides general comments, and sets forth the actions to be taken to address the GAO draft recommendations.

VA appreciates the opportunity to comment on your draft report.

Sincerely,
Peter M. O'Rourke
Chief of Staff

Enclosure

General Comments

The Veterans Health Administration (VHA) Office of Community Care (OCC) will work collaboratively with the VHA's Office of Veteran's Access to Care, Department of Veterans Affairs (VA) Office of Information and Technology, and other program offices to further evaluate modifications to the current wait-time goals and measurement processes enhancements that can be used to ensure comparability with VHA medical facilities.

VHA will be monitoring wait-times for all Veterans who use community care whether the care is provided by VHA's regional Community Care Network or by an individual community provider not included in the network. For the majority of appointment scheduling activities, however, VHA intends to be able to compare the wait-time performance of community-care providers against VHA medical facilities to ensure that Veterans receive timely care.

VHA will also monitor average drive times between Veterans' homes and the practice locations of community-care network providers to ensure that the contractors establish and maintain sufficient networks of qualified providers.

As VHA transitions to the Community Care Network (CCN) contracts, VA's medical centers (VAMCs) will have responsibility for scheduling Veterans' community-care appointments. VHA's OCC will utilize a combination of features inherent in the Computerized Patient Record System consult package and within the new referral and authorization system called Health Share Referral Manager (HSRM) to measure the time it takes to review and accept consults, prepare referrals, and schedule Veteran's community appointments. This capacity will exist whether the providers in the community are within the CCN or individual community providers.

VHA's new HSRM will support:

- Scheduling of community-care appointments for Veterans who will see a contracted regional network provider.
- Functionality to document the reason that a Veteran was not scheduled for the community-care appointment.
- Robust reporting function that will be able to support both VAMCs and national level reviews, including those for performance against wait-time goals.

HSRM will be a key component of an overall system that will facilitate the seamless, efficient information sharing among VAMCs, VHA clinicians, Third-Party Administrators (TPAs), community providers, and Veterans.

VHA is currently planning on 18 months to fully implement HSRM at all VAMCs beginning with the medical centers in Region 1, followed by Region 3, Region 2, and then Region 4 and the Pacific Islands. Deployment to pilot sites is anticipated by the end of September 2018.

By October 2018, OCC will complete the identification and design of these systems and components to facilitate seamless, efficient information sharing among VAMCs, VHA clinicians, TPAs, community providers, and Veterans. Additional time will be needed to fully implement and confirm viability of this system design.

VHA is in the process of evaluating the outcomes from the scheduling pilots conducted at the Alaska and Fargo VA Health Care Systems. The evaluation report to be completed will include a quantitative analysis of outcomes for Alaska and Fargo, North Dakota and will assess the timeliness of scheduling at each step of the piloted process.

Once VHA receives authority to consolidate community-care programs, VHA will ensure documentation of a future consolidated community care program will comply with VHA Directive 6330 titled *Controlled National Policy/Directives Management System* and the needs of the program office and field.

Recommendation 1

The Under Secretary for Health should establish an achievable wait-time goal for the consolidated community care program that VA plans to implement that will permit VHA to monitor whether veterans are receiving VA community care within time frames that are comparable to the amount of time they would otherwise wait to receive care at VHA medical facilities.

VA Comments

Concur

The Veterans Health Administration's (VHA) Office of Community Care (OCC) will work collaboratively with VHA's Office of Veteran's Access to Care (OVAC), Department of Veterans Affairs (VA) Office of Information and Technology (OI&T) and other VA Central Office (VACO) program offices to further evaluate modifications to the current wait-time goals and process enhancements to establish achievable wait time goals for the consolidated community-care program that can be monitored and compared to wait-time standards at VHA medical facilities.

OCC has established achievable wait-time goals for Veterans receiving care in the community consistent with internal VA scheduling and consult directives 1230 and 1232 for a significant population of Veterans receiving community care. However, currently those goals will be applied only when the initial request for community care comes from a VA provider directly to a facility community-care office, as opposed to when a consult is generated by a VA provider for VA care that is found not to be available within the requested timeframe and the Veteran opts in to community care. Those consults are forwarded to community care. These latter consults will not have a wait-time goal of the appointment occurring within 30 days of the

Clinically Indicated Date (CID), now called the Patient Indicated Date (PID), as is expected for appointments within VA or directly requested to a facility's community-care office. The forwarded consults will be measured against the time from when the request arrived in the facility community-care office to the time the appointment is made and then when the appointment occurs. The team working on a solution to support this recommendation will work to improve the appointment process or adjust appropriate goals to meet this recommendation.

For Consults Sent Directly to Facility's Office for Community Care	Receipt of Consult Request for Community Care to Created Appt.	Receipt of Consult Request for Community Care to Date of Scheduled Appt.	PID to-date of Scheduled Appt.
Wait-time Goals	14 days	30 days	< 30 days of PID
Ability to Measure	Yes	Yes	Yes
Wait-time goals	14 days	30 days	Not Yet Established
Ability to Measure	Yes	Yes	Yes

The status is in process with a target completion date of May 2019.

1/1-1A established the goals associated with the recommendation; however, full implementation is dependent on Community Care Network (CCN) contract award with an implementation timeframe expected to be complete by December 2019.

Recommendation 2

The Under Secretary for Health should design an appointment scheduling process for the consolidated community care program that VA plans to implement that sets forth time frames within which (1) veterans' referrals must be processed, (2) veterans' appointments must be scheduled, and (3) veterans' appointments must occur, which are consistent with the wait-time goal VHA has established for the program.

VA Comments

Concur

OCC will work collaboratively with OVAC, VA OI&T and other VACO program offices to design a scheduling process based upon achievable wait-time goals for the consolidated community-care program once the same reevaluated achievable wait-time goals for care received at VHA medical facilities and community care facilities are established.

VHA's OCC has established a thoughtfully designed scheduling process for once a consult reaches a facility's community-care office, but not for consults that were originally sent to a VHA internal clinic and then forwarded to community care.

Appointment scheduling standards for care in the community were also addressed in consult directive 1232* (B-10 &12) and to the Deputy Under Secretary for Health for Operations and Management memo, *Scheduling and Consult Policy Updates,* published June 5, 2017 (see Attachment). These scheduling standards are depicted in the chart outlined below.

Appointment Scheduling Standards

	Initiate Referral Processing	**Time to Schedule**	**Time to Appointment**
	Days from consult receipt in facility community-care office to initiate scheduling (see Attachment).	Days from consult receipt in facility community-care office to appointment scheduled.*	Days from consult receipt in facility community-care office to community appointment date CCN.*
Target Days from Community-Care Consult Entry	Within 2 days	Within 14 days	Within 30 days

VHA will be monitoring wait-times for all Veterans who use community care — whether the care is provided by a regional network or an individual community provider. VHA intends to be able to compare the wait-time performance of community-care providers against VHA medical facilities to ensure that Veterans receive timely care.

The status is in process with a target completion date of September 2019.

Recommendation 3

The Under Secretary for Health should establish a mechanism that will allow VHA to systematically monitor the average number of days it takes for VAMCs to prepare referrals, for VAMCs or TPAs to schedule veterans' appointments, and for veterans' appointments to occur, under the consolidated community care program that VA plans to implement.

VA Comments

Concur

As VHA transitions to the Community Care Network (CCN) contracts, staff at a facility's community-care office will be responsible for scheduling Veterans' community-care appointments. OCC will utilize a combination of features inherent in the Computerized Patient Record System (CPRS) consult package and features within the new referral and authorization system called Health Share Referral Manager (HSRM) to measure the time it takes to review and accept consults, prepare referrals and schedule Veterans community-care appointments. Reports will be made available for VHA and every VA medical center (VAMC) to review the average days to move from one step in the process to the next. Additionally, VHA will be able to drill down to the individual referral to understand every unique case. This capacity will exist whether the providers in the community are within the CCN or individual community providers. VHA is currently planning on 18 months to fully implement the HSRM system at all VAMCs beginning with the medical centers in Region 1, followed by Region 3, Region 2, and then Region 4 and the Pacific Islands. By December 2018, however, VHA will have designed and tested the system's capabilities relative to the recommendation. The status is in process with a target completion date of December 2018.

Recommendation 4

The Under Secretary for Health should implement a mechanism to prevent veterans' clinically indicated dates from being modified by individuals other than VHA clinicians when Veterans are referred to the consolidated community care program that VA plans to implement.

VA Comments

Concur

VA has implemented a mechanism to prevent CID, now called PID, from being modified by individuals other than VHA clinicians when Veterans are referred to the consolidated community-care program currently in place and is planning for future changes. Specifically, all requests to community care now come in the form of consults. Consult documents are created by VHA clinicians who must indicate the PID before they can sign the document.

Under the consolidated program, the referral process will be built off the consult document communicating the request to community care. Additionally, VHA has purchased a new referral and authorization system called HSRM. HSRM will accept the unalterable PID from the consult document in the process of creating the new referral to be sent to a community provider. VHA is currently planning on 18 months to fully implement this system at all VAMCs beginning with the medical centers in Region 1, followed by Region 3, Region 2, and then Region 4 and the Pacific Islands. By December 2018, however, VHA will have designed and tested the system's capabilities relative to the recommendation. The status is in process with a target completion date of December 2018.

Recommendation 5

The Under Secretary for Health should implement a mechanism to separate clinically urgent referrals and authorizations from those for which the VAMC or the TPA has decided to expedite appointment scheduling for administrative reasons.

VA Comments

Non-Concur

GAO's recommended solution is no longer needed because VHA has resolved the issue with the new CCN contract. Under the new CCN contract, facility community-care office staff will have responsibility for scheduling Veterans' community-care appointments with CCN providers, rather than the previous situation where administrators had to route referrals to the TPAs for scheduling.

With the implementation of VHA's CCN, VHA anticipates that there will no longer be a need to separate clinically urgent referrals from those that need expediting under this new approach,

Recommendation 6

The Under Secretary for Health should (1) establish oversight mechanisms to ensure that VHA is collecting reliable data on the reasons that VAMC or TPA staff are unsuccessful in scheduling Veterans' appointments through the consolidated community care program VA plans to implement and (2) demonstrate that it has corrected any identified deficiencies.

VA Comments

Concur

OCC recently purchased a Referral and Authorization commercial off-the-shelf product named HSRM. HSRM, in combination with CPRS documentation graphical user-interface consult toolbox, will support the scheduling of community care and will provide the functionality to document the reason why a Veteran was unable to be scheduled for a community-care appointment. These products will have robust reporting functions that will allow for both VAMC and national monitoring of the frequency that community-care appointments are unsuccessfully scheduled and the reasons behind the inability to schedule.

OCC will collaborate with all other applicable national VA program offices to ensure that clear policies and procedures are in place for employees who use these tools and that local, regional, and national oversight and monitoring processes are in place. Oversight mechanisms will include auditing and testing to ensure compliance with the use of these tools and that appropriate corrective actions are taken when deficiencies in the scheduling process are identified. The status is in process with a target completion date of April 2019.

Recommendation 7

The Secretary for Veterans Affairs should ensure that the contracts for the consolidated community care program VA plans to implement include performance metrics that will allow VHA to monitor average driving times between veterans' homes and the practice locations of community providers that participate in the TPA's networks.

VA Comments

Concur

VHA intends that Veterans have access to contracted CCN providers within a reasonable driving time from their home. VHA also expects to be able to monitor average drive times between Veterans' homes and the practice locations of providers in the CCN.

VHA's CCN Request for Proposal (RFP) for Regions 1, 2, and 3 specifies that the contractor must provide and maintain a comprehensive network of qualified healthcare providers and practitioners that extends across the entirety of each CCN Region. This network must be sufficient in number and types of providers, practitioners and facilities to ensure that all services set forth in the contract are accessible within VHA-defined timeframes. The RFP further defines maximum drive-time requirements in both the Performance Work Statement and Quality Assurance Plan (QASP). Section 3.6 (Network Adequacy Management) of the RFP specifically indicates that the Contractor must monitor their performance against the following Veteran drive times:

CCN RFP: Maximum Drive Times

Drive Times	
Primary Care	
Urban	Thirty (30) minutes
Rural	Forty-five (45) minutes
Highly Rural Location	Sixty (60) minutes
General Care	
Urban	Forty-five (45) minutes
Rural	One hundred (100) minutes
Highly Rural Location	One hundred eighty (180) minutes
Complementary and Integrative Healthcare Services (CIHS)	
Urban	Forty-five (45) minutes
Rural	One hundred (100) minutes
Highly Rural Location	One hundred eighty (180) minutes

In addition, the Contractor will be required to provide VHA with a Network Adequacy Performance Report, with the following:

i. average drive time, calculated per claim received and calculated using Bing Maps or other geo-mapping utility approved by VA based on the distance between Veteran address maintained in the eligibility data and the rendering provider's physical address without factoring in allocations for traffic conditions.

ii. average appointment availability to evaluate wait times, calculated using the date the referral is sent to provider from VA and actual appointment date on the first claim associated with that referral.

iii. any further analysis that takes into consideration any rescheduled, cancelled, or missed appointments and/or Veteran or CCN provider complaint data received regarding drive time or appointment availability standards.

iv. any gaps in network adequacy for average drive time and appointment availability, categorized by health care service category and geographic location to include an Urban, Rural, or Highly Rural Location indicator and documentation of rescheduled, cancelled, or missed appointments.

The QASP describes the systematic methods used to monitor performance and provides a means for evaluating whether the contractor is meeting the performance standards/quality levels identified in the performance work statement. The standards/ Acceptable Quality Levels for geographic accessibility to a provider based on drive times for Primary Care, General Care and Complementary and Integrative Health Services (CIHS) are as follows:

Outstanding — 97 percent and above
Very Good - 96.9 percent — 95 percent
Good - 94.99 percent — 90 percent
Marginal - 89.9 percent and below

If the Contractor has not met the minimum requirements, it may be asked to develop a corrective action plan to show how and by what date it intends to bring performance up to the required levels. The Contractor will provide monthly and quarterly reports, and will meet with OCC and other relevant government personnel during a quarterly Performance Management Review to review these reports and any Corrective Action Plans, address issues and concerns of both parties, discuss projected outlook for improved efficiency and effectiveness, and any other programmatic or performance concerns. Performance metrics for Region 4 and the Pacific Islands will be established when the RFP is published, currently expected to be in the first quarter of fiscal year 2019. The status is in process with a target completion date of December 2018.

Recommendation 8

The Secretary of Veterans Affairs should establish a system for the consolidated community care program VA plans to implement to help facilitate seamless, efficient information sharing among VAMCs, VHA clinicians, TPAs, community providers, and veterans. Specifically, this system should allow all of these entities to electronically exchange information for the purposes of care coordination.

VA Comments

Concur

OCC recently purchased a Referral and Authorization commercial off-the-shelf product named HSRM. HSRM will be a key component of an overall system that will facilitate the seamless, efficient information sharing among VAMCs, VHA clinicians, TPAs, community providers, and Veterans.

For example: VAMC community-care staff will assign the referral in HSRM, including appropriate medical documentation, to the community-care provider. The community-care provider will review the request in HRSM and determine to accept or reject the referral. If the community-care provider accepts the referral, they will document the appointment date in HRSM and then follow-up with uploading medical records in HSRM after treatment is completed. This bidirectional communication will assist in care coordination for the Veteran.

Veterans will receive communications for VA through telephone, MyHealtheVet secured messaging where appropriate and acceptable, and the VA online scheduling application where appropriate and acceptable. They will also use the VA website to search for community providers in the network. All of the systems and processes will be referenced in the OCC's transition guidebook by October 2018.

VHA is currently planning on 18 months to fully implement HSRM at all VAMCs beginning with the medical centers in Region 1, followed by Region 3, Region 2, and then Region **4** and the Pacific Islands. By December 2018, however, VHA will have designed and tested the system's capabilities relative to the recommendation. The status is in process with a target completion date of December 2018.

Recommendation 9

The Under Secretary for Health should conduct a comprehensive evaluation of the outcomes of the two appointment scheduling pilots it established at the Alaska and Fargo VA Health Care Systems (where VAMC staff, rather than TPA staff, are responsible for scheduling veterans' Choice

Program appointments), which should include a comparison of the timeliness with which VAMC staff and TPA staff completed each step of the Choice Program appointment scheduling process, as well as the overall timeliness with which veterans received appointments.

VA Comments

Concur

VHA is in the process of evaluating the outcomes from the scheduling pilots conducted at the Alaska and Fargo VA Health Care Systems. The evaluation report to be completed will include a quantitative analysis of outcomes for Alaska and Fargo, North Dakota, and will assess the timeliness of scheduling at each step of the piloted process. The status is in process with a target completion date of July 2018.

Recommendation 10

The Under Secretary for Health should issue a comprehensive policy directive and operations manual for the consolidated community care program VA plans to implement and ensure that these documents are reviewed and updated in a timely manner after any significant changes to the program occur.

VA Comments

Concur in principle

VHA concurs in principle because documentation of a future consolidated community-care program will comply with VHA Directive 6330, *Controlled National Policy/Directives Management System,* and the needs of the program office and field. These documents may take many forms, such as, standard operating procedures, toolkits, or other guidance. VHA has found that premature issuance of new policy directives or operational manuals can create more confusion rather than clarity and may not be the most optimal solution for ensuring consistent implementation nationwide. Management will consider whether new policy directives are needed after the CCN contract has been fully implemented and interim challenges to implementation have been resolved. The status is in process with a target completion date of December 2019.

APPENDIX VIII: ACCESSIBLE DATA

Data Table

Accessible Data for Figure 7: Comparison of Processes for Arranging Choice Program and Individually Authorized Department of Veterans Affairs (VA) Community Care

n/a	Steps for time-eligible veterans to obtain Choice Program care[a]	Steps for veterans to obtain individually authorized VA community care
Authorization process	1. VA clinician determines veteran needs care. 2. VAMC verifies services unavailable through VA or a facility with which VA has a sharing agreement and veteran is eligible for Choice Program care. 3. VAMC staff contact veteran and confirm they want Choice Program care. 4. VAMC staff upload referral for Choice Program care to TPA's portal. 5. TPA reviews and accepts referral. 6. TPA calls veteran three times to confirm they want Choice Program care. If veteran not reached, TPA sends letter and awaits veteran's response.	1. VA clinician determines veteran needs care. 2. VAMC verifies services are unavailable through VA or a facility with which VA has a sharing agreement and veteran is eligible for community care. 3. VAMC creates community care authorization and selects community provider.
Appointment scheduling	7. TPA contacts community provider(s) and schedules veteran's appointment. 8. TPA contacts veteran to confirm appointment. 9. Veteran attends appointment.	4. VAMC calls veteran twice to select a provider and schedule appointment. If veteran is not reached by phone, VAMC mails a letter to the veteran and requests that the veteran contact the VAMC to schedule an appointment with a community provider. 5. VAMC sends letter with appointment information to veteran. 6. Veteran attends appointment.

n/a	Steps for time-eligible veterans to obtain Choice Program care[a]	Steps for veterans to obtain individually authorized VA community care
Record retrieval and follow up	10. TPA obtains medical documentation from community provider, confirming appointment attended. 11. TPA uploads medical documentation and enters appointment information into its portal. 12. VAMC retrieves medical documentation from TPA portal and scans it into veteran's VA electronic health record.	7. VAMC contacts veteran to confirm appointment attended. 8. VAMC obtains medical documentation from community provider and scans it into veteran's VA electronic health record.

Legend: TPA=third party administrator; VAMC=VA medical center.

AGENCY COMMENT LETTER

Accessible Text for Appendix VII: Comments from the Department of Veteran's Affairs

DEPARTMENT OF VETERANS AFFAIRS
WASHINGTON DC 20420
May 16, 2018
Ms. A. Nicole Clowers
Managing Director
Health Care
U.S. Government Accountability Office

Dear Ms. Clowers:

The Department of Veterans Affairs (VA) has reviewed the Government Accountability Office's (GAO) draft report, "VETERANS CHOICE PROGRAM: Improvements Needed to Address Access-Related Challenges as VA Plans Consolidation of its Community Care Programs" (GAO-18-281).

The enclosure provides general comments, and sets forth the actions to be taken to address the GAO draft recommendations.

VA appreciates the opportunity to comment on your draft report. Sincerely,

Peter M. O'Rourke

Chief of Staff

Enclosure

Department of Veterans Affairs (VA) Comments to Government Accountability Office (GAO) Draft Report "VETERANS CHOICE **PROGRAM: Improvements Needed to Address Access- Related Challenges as VA Plans Consolidation of its Community Care Programs**" (GAO-18-281)

General Comments:

The Veterans Health Administration (VHA) Office of Community Care (OCC) will work collaboratively with the VHA's Office of Veteran's Access to Care, Department of Veterans Affairs (VA) Office of Information and Technology, and other program offices to further evaluate modifications to the current wait-time goals and measurement processes enhancements that can be used to ensure comparability with VHA medical facilities.

VHA will be monitoring wait-times for all Veterans who use community care whether the care is provided by VHA's regional Community Care Network or by an individual community provider not included in the network. For the majority of appointment scheduling activities, however, VHA intends to be able to compare the wait-lime performance of community-care providers against VHA medical facilities to ensure that Veterans receive timely care.

VHA will also monitor average drive times between Veterans' homes and the practice locations of community-care network providers to ensure that the contractors establish and maintain sufficient networks of qualified providers.

As VHA transitions to the Community Care Network (CCN) contracts, VA's medical centers (VAMCs) will have responsibility for scheduling Veterans' community-care appointments. VHA's OCC will utilize a combination of features inherent in the Computerized Patient Record System consult package and within the new referral and authorization system called Health Share Referral Manager (HSRM) to measure the time it takes to review and accept consults, prepare referrals, and schedule Veteran's community appointments. This capacity will exist whether the providers in the community are within the CCN or individual community providers.

VHA's new HSRM will support:

- Scheduling of community-care appointments for Veterans who will see a contracted regional network provider.
- Functionality to document the reason that a Veteran was not scheduled for the community-care appointment.
- Robust reporting function that will be able to support both VAMCs and national level reviews, including those for performance against wait-time goals.

HSRM will be a key component of an overall system that will facilitate the seamless, efficient information sharing among VAMCs, VHA clinicians, Third-Party Administrators (TPAs), community providers, and Veterans.

VHA is currently planning on 18 months to fully implement HSRM at all VAMCs beginning with the medical centers in Region 1, followed by Region 3, Region 2, and then Region 4 and the Pacific Islands. Deployment to pilot sites is anticipated by the end of September 2018.

By October 2018, OCC will complete the identification and design of these systems and components to facilitate seamless, efficient information sharing among VAMCs, VHA clinicians, TPAs, community providers, and Veterans. Additional time will be needed to fully implement and confirm viability of this system design.

VHA is in the process of evaluating the outcomes from the scheduling pilots conducted at the Alaska and Fargo VA Health Care Systems. The evaluation report to be completed will include a quantitative analysis of outcomes for Alaska and Fargo, North Dakota and will assess the timeliness of scheduling at each step of the piloted process.

Once VHA receives authority to consolidate community-care programs, VHA will ensure documentation of a future consolidated community-care program will comply with VHA Directive 6330 titled *Controlled National Policy/Directives Management System* and the needs of the program office and field.

Recommendation 1

The Under Secretary for Health should establish an achievable wait-time goal for the consolidated community care program that VA plans to implement that will permit VHA to monitor whether veterans are receiving VA community care within time frames that are comparable to the amount of time they would otherwise wait to receive care at VHA medical facilities.

VA Comments

Concur

The Veterans Health Administration's (VHA) Office of Community Care (OGG) will work collaboratively with VHA's Office of Veteran's Access to Care (OVAC), Department of Veterans Affairs (VA) Office of Information and Technology (01&T) and other VA Central Office (VACO) program offices to further evaluate modifications to the current wait-time goals and process enhancements to establish achievable wait time goals for the consolidated community-care program that can be monitored and compared to wait-time standards at VHA medical facilities.

OGG has established achievable wait-time goals for Veterans receiving care in the community consistent with internal VA scheduling and consult directives 1230 and 1232 for a significant population of Veterans receiving community care. However, currently those goals will be applied only when the initial request for community care comes from a VA provider directly to a facility community-care office, as opposed to when a consult is generated by a VA provider for VA care that is found not to be available within the requested timeframe and the Veteran opts in to community care. Those consults are forwarded to community care. These latter consults will not have a wait-time goal of the appointment occurring within 30 days of the

Clinically Indicated Date (CID), now called the Patient Indicated Date (PIO), as is expected for appointments within VA or directly requested to a facility's community-care office. The forwarded consults will be measured against the time from when the request arrived in the facility community-care office to the time the appointment is made and then when the appointment occurs. The team working on a solution to support this recommendation will work to improve the appointment process or adjust appropriate goals to meet this recommendation.

For Consults Sent Directly to Facility's Office for Community Care	Receipt of Consult Request for Community Care to Created Appt.	Receipt of Consult Request for Community Care to Date of Scheduled Appt.	PID to-date of Scheduled Appt.
Wait-time Goals	14 days	30 days	< 30 days of PID
Ability to Measure	Yes	Yes	Yes
Wait-time goals	14 days	30 days	Not Yet Established
Ability to Measure	Yes	Yes	Yes

The status is in process with a target completion date of May 2019.

*VHA established the goals associated with the recommendation; however, full implementation is dependent on Community Care Network (CCN) contract award with an implementation timeframe expected to be complete by December 2019.

Recommendation 2

The Under Secretary for Health should design an appointment scheduling process for the consolidated community care program that VA plans to implement that sets forth time frames within which (1) veterans' referrals must be processed, (2) veterans' appointments must be scheduled, and (3) veterans' appointments must occur, which are consistent with the wait-time goal VHA has established for the program.

VA Comments

Concur

OCC will work collaboratively with OVAC, VA OI&T and other VACO program offices to design a scheduling process based upon achievable wait-time goals for the consolidated community-care program once the same reevaluated achievable wait-time goals for care received at VHA medical facilities and community care facilities are established.

VHA's OCC has established a thoughtfully designed scheduling process for once a consult reaches a facility's community-care office, but not for consults that were originally sent to a VHA internal clinic and then forwarded to community care.

Appointment scheduling standards for care in the community were also addressed in consult directive 1232* (B-1O & 12) and to the Deputy Under Secretary for Health for Operations and Management memo, Scheduling and Consult Policy Updates, published June 5, 2017. These scheduling standards are depicted in the chart outlined below.

VHA will be monitoring wait-times for all Veterans who use community care - whether the care is provided by a regional network or an individual community provider. VHA intends to be able to compare the wait-time performance of community-care providers against VHA medical facilities to ensure that Veterans receive timely care.

The status is in process with a target completion date of September 2019.

VA Comments

Concur

As VHA transitions to the Community Care Network (CCN) contracts, staff at a facility's community-care office will be responsible for scheduling Veterans' community-care appointments. OCC will utilize a combination of features inherent in the Computerized Patient Record System (CPRS)

Appointment Scheduling Standards

n/a	Initiate Referral Processing	Time to Schedule	Time to Appointment
n/a	Days from consult receipt in facility community-care office to initiate scheduling (see Attachment).	Days from consult receipt in facility community-care office to appointment scheduled.*	Days from consult receipt in facility community-care office to community appointment date CCN.*
Target Days from Community-Care Consult Entry	Within 2 days	Within 14 days	Within 30 days

consult package and features within the new referral and authorization system called Health Share Referral Manager (HSRM) to measure the time it takes to review and accept consults, prepare referrals and schedule Veterans community-care appointments. Reports will be made available for VHA and every VA medical center (VAMC) to review the average days to move from one step in the process to the next. Additionally, VHA will be able to drill down to the individual referral to understand every unique case. This capacity will exist whether the providers in the community are within the CCN or individual community providers. VHA is currently planning on 18 months to fully implement the HSRM system at all VAMCs beginning with the medical centers in Region 1, followed by Region 3, Region 2, and then Region 4 and the Pacific Islands. By December 2018, however,

VHA will have designed and tested the system's capabilities relative to the recommendation. The status is in process with a target completion date of December 2018.

Recommendation 4

The Under Secretary for Health should implement a mechanism to prevent veterans' clinically indicated dates from being modified by individuals other than VHA clinicians when Veterans are referred to the consolidated community care program that VA plans to implement.

VA Comments

Concur

VA has implemented a mechanism to prevent CID, now called PID, from being modified by individuals other than VHA clinicians when Veterans are referred to the consolidated community-care program currently in place and is planning for future changes. Specifically, all requests to community care now come in the form of consults. Consult documents are created by VHA clinicians who must indicate the PID before they can sign the document.

Under the consolidated program, the referral process will be built off the consult document communicating the request to community care. Additionally, VHA has purchased a new referral and authorization system called HSRM. HSRM will accept the unalterable PID from the consult document in the process of creating the new referral to be sent to a community provider. VHA is currently planning on 18 months to fully implement this system at all VAMCs beginning with the medical centers in Region 1, followed by Region 3, Region 2, and then Region 4 and the Pacific Islands. By December 2018, however, VHA will have designed and tested the system's capabilities relative to the recommendation. The status is in process with a target completion date of December 2018.

Recommendation 5

The Under Secretary for Health should implement a mechanism to separate clinically urgent referrals and authorizations from those for which the VAMC or the TPA has decided to expedite appointment scheduling for administrative reasons.

VA Comments

Non-Concur

GAO's recommended solution is no longer needed because VHA has resolved the issue with the new CCN contract. Under the new CCN contract, facility community-care office staff will have responsibility for scheduling

Veterans' community-care appointments with CCN providers, rather than the previous situation where administrators had to route referrals to the TPAs for scheduling.

With the implementation of VHA's CCN, VHA anticipates that there will no longer be a need to separate clinically urgent referrals from those that need expediting under this new approach.

Recommendation 6

The Under Secretary for Health should (1) establish oversight mechanisms to ensure that VHA is collecting reliable data on the reasons that VAMC or TPA staff are unsuccessful in scheduling Veterans' appointments through the consolidated community care program VA plans to implement and (2) demonstrate that it has corrected any identified deficiencies.

VA Comments

Concur

OCC recently purchased a Referral and Authorization commercial off-the-shelf product named HSRM. HSRM, in combination with CPRS documentation graphical user-interface consult toolbox, will support the scheduling of community care and will provide the functionality to document the reason why a Veteran was unable to be scheduled for a community-care appointment. These products will have robust reporting functions that will allow for both VAMC and national monitoring of the frequency that community-care appointments are unsuccessfully scheduled and the reasons behind the inability to schedule.

OCC will collaborate with all other applicable national VA program offices to ensure that clear policies and procedures are in place for employees who use these tools and that local, regional, and national oversight and monitoring processes are in place. Oversight mechanisms will include auditing and testing to ensure compliance with the use of these tools and that appropriate corrective actions are taken when deficiencies in the scheduling process are identified. The status is in process with a target completion date of April 2019.

Recommendation 7

The Secretary for Veterans Affairs should ensure that the contracts for the consolidated community care program VA plans to implement include performance metrics that will allow VHA to monitor average driving times between veterans' homes and the practice locations of community providers that participate in the TPA's networks.

VA Comments

Concur

VHA intends that Veterans have access to contracted CCN providers within a reasonable driving time from their home. VHA also expects to be able to monitor average drive times between Veterans' homes and the practice locations of providers in the CCN.

VHA's CCN Request for Proposal (RFP) for Regions 1, 2, and 3 specifies that the contractor must provide and maintain a comprehensive network of qualified healthcare providers and practitioners that extends across the entirety of each CCN Region. This network must be sufficient in number and types of providers, practitioners and facilities to ensure that all services set forth in the contract are accessible within VHA-defined timeframes. The RFP further defines maximum drive-time requirements in both the Performance Work Statement and Quality Assurance Plan (QASP). Section 3.6

(Network Adequacy Management) of the RFP specifically indicates that the Contractor must monitor their performance against the following Veteran drive times:

CCN RFP: Maximum Drive Times

Drive Times		
Primary Care	Urban	Thirty (30) minutes
Primary Care	Rural	Forty-five (45) minutes
Primary Care	Highly Rural Location	Sixty (60) minutes
General Care	Urban	Forty-five (45) minutes
General Care	Rural	One hundred (100) minutes
General Care	Highly Rural Location	One hundred eighty(180)minutes
Complementary and Integrative Healthcare Services (CIHS)	Urban	Forty-five (45) minutes
Complementary and Integrative Healthcare Services (CIHS)	Rural	One hundred (100) minutes
Complementary and Integrative Healthcare Services (CIHS)	Highly Rural Location	One hundred eighty(180) minutes

In addition, the Contractor will be required to provide VHA with a Network Adequacy Performance Report, with the following:

i. average drive time, calculated per claim received and calculated using Bing Maps or other gee-mapping utility approved by VA based on the distance between Veteran address maintained in the eligibility data and the rendering provider's physical address without factoring in allocations for traffic conditions.

ii. average appointment availability to evaluate wait times, calculated using the date the referral is sent to provider from VA and actual appointment date on the first claim associated with that referral.

iii. any further analysis that takes into consideration any rescheduled, cancelled, or missed appointments and/or Veteran or CCN provider complaint data received regarding drive time or appointment availability standards.

iv. any gaps in network adequacy for average drive time and appointment availability, categorized by health care service category and geographic location to include an Urban, Rural, or Highly Rural Location indicator and documentation of rescheduled, cancelled, or missed appointments.

The QASP describes the systematic methods used to monitor performance and provides a means for evaluating whether the contractor is meeting the performance standards/quality levels identified in the performance work statement. The standards/ Acceptable Quality Levels for geographic accessibility to a provider based on drive times for Primary Care, General Care and Complementary and Integrative Health Services (CIHS) are as follows:

- Outstanding - 97 percent and above
- Very Good - 96.9 percent - 95 percent
- Good - 94.99 percent - 90 percent
- Marginal - 89.9 percent and below

If the Contractor has not met the minimum requirements, it may be asked to develop a corrective action plan to show how and by what date it intends to bring performance up to the required levels. The Contractor will provide monthly and quarterly reports, and will meet with OCC and other relevant government personnel during a quarterly Performance Management Review to review these reports and any Corrective Action Plans, address issues and concerns of both parties, discuss projected outlook for improved efficiency and effectiveness, and any other programmatic or performance concerns. Performance metrics for Region 4 and the Pacific Islands will be established when the RFP is published, currently expected to be in the first quarter of fiscal year 2019. The status is in process with a target completion date of December 2018.

Recommendation 8

The Secretary of Veterans Affairs should establish a system for the consolidated community care program VA plans to implement to help facilitate seamless, efficient information sharing among VAMCs, VHA clinicians, TPAs, community providers, and veterans. Specifically, this system should allow all of these entities to electronically exchange information for the purposes of care coordination.

VA Comments

Concur

OCC recently purchased a Referral and Authorization commercial off-the-shelf product named HSRM. HSRM will be a key component of an overall system that will facilitate the seamless, efficient information sharing among VAMCs, VHA clinicians, TPAs, community providers, and Veterans.

For example: VAMC community-care staff will assign the referral in HSRM, including appropriate medical documentation, to the community-care provider. The community- care provider will review the request in HRSM and determine to accept or reject the referral. If the community-care provider accepts the referral, they will document the appointment date in HRSM and then follow-up with uploading medical records in HSRM

After treatment is completed. This bidirectional communication will assist in care coordination for the Veteran.

Veterans will receive communications for VA through telephone, MyHealtheVet secured messaging where appropriate and acceptable, and the VA online scheduling application where appropriate and acceptable. They will also use the VA website to search for community providers in the network. All of the systems and processes will be referenced in the OCC's transition guidebook by October 2018.

VHA is currently planning on 18 months to fully implement HSRM at all VAMCs beginning with the medical centers in Region 1, followed by Region 3, Region 2, and then Region 4 and the Pacific Islands. By December 2018, however, VHA will have designed and tested the system's capabilities relative to the recommendation. The status is in process with a target completion date of December 2018.

Recommendation 9

The Under Secretary for Health should conduct a comprehensive evaluation of the outcomes of the two appointment scheduling pilots it established at the Alaska and Fargo VA Health Care Systems (where VAMC staff, rather than TPA staff, are responsible for scheduling veterans' Choice

Program appointments), which should include a comparison of the timeliness with which VAMC staff and TPA staff completed each step of the Choice Program appointment scheduling process, as well as the overall timeliness with which veterans received appointments.

VA Comments

Concur

VHA is in the process of evaluating the outcomes from the scheduling pilots conducted at the Alaska and Fargo VA Health Care Systems. The evaluation report to be completed will include a quantitative analysis of outcomes for Alaska and Fargo, North Dakota, and will assess the timeliness of scheduling at each step of the piloted process. The status is in process with a target completion date of July 2018.

Recommendation 10

The Under Secretary for Health should issue a comprehensive policy directive and operations manual for the consolidated community care program VA plans to implement and ensure that these documents are reviewed and updated in a timely manner after any significant changes to the program occur.

VA Comments

Concur in Principle

VHA concurs in principle because documentation of a future consolidated community-care program will comply with VHA Directive 6330, Controlled National Policy/Directives Management System, and the needs of the program office and field. These documents may take many forms, such as, standard operating procedures, toolkits, or other guidance. VHA has found that premature issuance of new policy directives or operational manuals can create more confusion rather than clarity and may not be the most optimal solution for ensuring consistent implementation nationwide. Management will consider whether new policy directives are needed after the CCN contract has been fully implemented and interim challenges to implementation have been resolved. The status is in process with a target completion date of December 2019.

In: The Veterans Choice Program (VCP)   ISBN: 978-1-53614-819-0
Editor: Mabel Page   © 2019 Nova Science Publishers, Inc.

Chapter 4

VETERANS CHOICE PROGRAM: FURTHER IMPROVEMENTS NEEDED TO HELP ENSURE TIMELY PAYMENTS TO COMMUNITY PROVIDERS[*]

United States Government Accountability Office

ABBREVIATIONS

OIG	Office of Inspector General
RFP	request for proposals
SAR	secondary authorization request
TPA	third-party administrator
VA	Department of Veterans Affairs

---

[*] This is an edited, reformatted and augmented version of United States Government Accountability Office Report to the Ranking Member of the Committee on Veterans' Affairs, U.S. Senate. Publication No. GAO-18-671, dated September 2018.

WHY GAO DID THIS STUDY

Questions have been raised about the lack of timeliness of TPAs' payments to community providers under the Choice Program and how this may affect the willingness of providers to participate in the program as well as in the forthcoming Veterans Community Care Program. You asked GAO to review issues related to the timeliness of TPAs' payments to community providers under the Choice Program.

This report examines, among other things, (1) the length of time TPAs have taken to pay community providers' claims and factors affecting timeliness of payments, and (2) actions taken by VA and the TPAs to reduce the length of time TPAs take to pay community providers for Choice Program claims.

GAO reviewed TPA data on the length of time taken to pay community provider claims from November 2014 through June 2018, the most recent data available at the time of GAO's review. GAO also reviewed documentation, such as the contracts between VA and its TPAs, and interviewed VA and TPA officials. In addition, GAO interviewed a non-generalizable sample of 15 community providers, selected based on their large Choice Program claims volume, to learn about their experiences with payment timeliness.

WHAT GAO RECOMMENDS

GAO is making two recommendations, including that VA should collect data on and monitor compliance with its requirements pertaining to customer service for community providers. VA concurred with GAO's recommendations and described steps it will take to implement them.

WHAT GAO FOUND

The Department of Veterans Affairs' (VA) Veterans Choice Program (Choice Program) was created in 2014 to address problems with veterans' timely access to care at VA medical facilities. The Choice Program allows eligible veterans to obtain health care services from providers not directly employed by VA (community providers), who are then reimbursed for their services through one of the program's two third-party administrators (TPA). GAO's analysis of TPA data available for November 2014 through June 2018 shows that the length of time the TPAs took to pay community providers' clean claims each month varied widely—from 7 days to 68 days. VA and its TPAs identified several key factors affecting timeliness of payments to community providers under the Choice Program, including VA's untimely payments to TPAs, which in turn extended the length of time TPAs took to pay community providers' claims; and inadequate provider education on filing claims.

Median Number of Days to Pay Clean Claims through VA's Third Party Administrators (TPA), November 2014 through June 2018

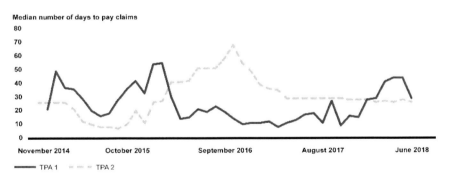

Source: GAO analysis of TPA data. | GAO-18-671.

VA has taken actions to address key factors that have contributed to the length of time TPAs have taken to pay community providers. For example, VA updated its payment system and related processes to pay TPAs more quickly. According to VA data, as of July 2018, VA was paying at least 90 percent of the TPAs' invoices within 7 days. In addition, VA and the TPAs have taken steps to improve provider education to help providers resolve claims processing issues. However, 9 of the 15 providers GAO interviewed said they continue to experience lengthy telephone hold times. According to VA and TPA officials, steps have been taken to improve the customer service offered to community providers. However, VA officials do not collect data on or monitor TPA compliance with customer service requirements—such as calls being answered within 30 seconds or less—for provider calls because they said they are not enforcing the requirements and are allowing TPAs to prioritize calls from veterans. Without collecting data and monitoring compliance, VA does not have information on challenges providers may face when contacting TPAs to resolve payment issues.

* * *

September 28, 2018
The Honorable Jon Tester Ranking Member
Committee on Veterans' Affairs United States Senate

Dear Senator Tester:

The Veterans Access, Choice, and Accountability Act of 2014 created the Veterans Choice Program (Choice Program) to address problems with veterans' timely access to care at Department of Veterans Affairs (VA) medical facilities.[1] Under the Choice Program, when eligible veterans face long wait times, lengthy travel distances, or other challenges accessing care at VA medical facilities, they may obtain health care services from community providers—that is, providers who are not directly employed by VA. The program is primarily administered by two contractors, known as third-party administrators (TPA)—TriWest Healthcare Alliance (TriWest) and Health Net Federal Services (Health Net)—which are responsible for, among other things, establishing nationwide networks of community

---

[1] Pub. L. No. 113-146, 128 Stat. 1754 (2014).

providers, scheduling appointments for veterans, and paying community providers for their services.

Since its implementation, the Choice Program has faced challenges and drawn scrutiny. External reviews, media reports, and congressional hearings held over the course of the Choice Program's implementation and operation have highlighted several programmatic weaknesses. These weaknesses have included insufficient community provider networks, significant delays in scheduling appointments, and a lack of timely payments by the TPAs to community providers.[2] Media reports suggest that the untimely payments to community providers have created financial hardship for some and a reluctance to continue participating in the Choice Program.[3] This has raised concerns that a reduction in participating community providers will increase wait times for veterans and result in longer travel distances, especially in rural areas. Due to these and other concerns, we concluded that VA health care is a high-risk area and added it to our High Risk List in 2015.[4]

Congress recently passed legislation to help address some of the challenges faced by the Choice Program and VA's other community care programs.[5] Specifically, the VA MISSION Act of 2018, signed into law in

---

[2] See, for example, Department of Veterans Affairs Office of Inspector General, Veterans Health Administration: Audit of the Timeliness and Accuracy of Choice Payments Processed Through the Fee Basis Claims System, Report No. 15-03036-47 (Washington, D.C.: Dec. 21, 2017); Quil Lawrence, Eric Whitney, and Michael Tomsic, "Despite $10B 'Fix,' Veterans Are Waiting Even Longer To See Doctors." Morning Edition (NPR, May 16, 2016) accessed January 27, 2017, http://w w w.npr.org/sections/health-shots/2016/05/16/477814218/ attempted-fix-for-va-healt h-delays-creates-new-bureaucracy; and Lee Romney, "Veterans Choice is Flawed, but Congress Is Stymied on a Solution," The Center for Investigative Reporting, (September 28, 2016, accessed January 27, 2017), https://w ww.revealnew s.org/article/veterans-choice-is-flawed-but-congress-is-stymied-ona-solution.

[3] See, for example, Stephanie Earls, "Veterans, Doctors Alike Stranded as Vet Choice Fails to Pay Its Bills," *The Gazette,* Mar. 17, 2018, accessed June 22, 2018, https://gazette.com/ health/veterans-doctors-alike-stranded-as-vet-choice-fails-to-pay-itsbills/article/1622450; and Nick Ochsner, "Slow VA Choice Authorization, Reimbursements Frustrate Doctors' Offices" (Mar. 22, 2016), accessed July 10, 2018.

[4] GAO, High-Risk Series: An Update, GAO-15-290 (Washington, D.C.: Feb. 11, 2015). GAO maintains a high-risk program to focus attention on government operations that it identifies as high risk due to their greater vulnerabilities to fraud, waste, abuse, and mismanagement or the need for transformation to address economy, efficiency, or effectiveness challenges.

[5] The Choice Program is one of several VA programs that facilitate care for veterans from community providers. For more information about these VA community care programs, including differences in eligibility requirements and payment rates, see GAO, *Veterans'*

June 2018, requires VA to consolidate the Choice Program and its other VA community care programs into one community care program—the Veterans Community Care Program—in addition to authorizing VA to utilize a TPA for claims processing and requiring VA to reimburse community providers in a timely manner.[6] Currently, VA is in the process of evaluating proposals for the Veterans Community Care Program. Under the current request for proposals (RFP) there will be an up to 1- year implementation period, and the new program is expected to begin serving veterans in fiscal year 2019. The Choice Program is expected to continue until that time and will statutorily sunset after June 6, 2019.

You asked us to review issues related to the timeliness of TPAs' payments to community providers under the Choice Program. In this report, we examine

1. the length of time TPAs have taken to pay community providers' claims under the Choice Program, VA's efforts to monitor these time frames, and factors that affected timeliness of payments, and
2. actions taken by VA and the TPAs to reduce the length of time TPAs take to pay community providers for Choice Program claims.

To examine the length of time TPAs have taken to pay community providers' claims under the Choice Program, factors affecting timeliness of payments, and VA's efforts to monitor these time frames, we reviewed TPA data on the length of time it took TPAs to pay claims and the number and percentage of claims rejected or denied over the course of the Choice Program, from November 2014 through June 2018, the most recent data available at the time of our review.[7] To assess the reliability of these data, we collected information from TPA officials regarding the reliability of the

---

Health Care: Proper Plan Needed to Modernize System for Paying Community Providers, GAO-16-353 (Washington, D.C.: May 11, 2016).

[6] Pub. L.No. 115-182, tit. I, 132 Stat. 182 (2018).

[7] According to TPA officials, rejected claims are claims returned up front to providers due to, for example, the use of invalid claim forms and missing provider identification numbers. Denied claims are claims that contain the necessary data elements but do not pass required claim processing steps, which, for example, verify the veteran's eligibility for the Choice Program and that a valid authorization for care is on file.

data and reviewed the data for obvious errors and missing values. We discussed and worked with TPA officials to resolve any identified data issues. On the basis of these steps, we determined the claim payment data were sufficiently reliable for the purposes of our reporting objectives. However, data limitations prohibited us from assessing the extent to which the two TPAs rejected or denied claims. We also reviewed VA and TPA documentation, such as the contracts between VA and its TPAs, contract modifications, and VA's RFP for its new contracts for the Veterans Community Care Program.[8] We interviewed VA contracting officials and officials from the Office of Community Care (the office within VA's Veterans Health Administration responsible for implementing and overseeing the Choice Program) as well as TPA officials about VA's efforts to monitor TPA data on payment time frames, as well as claim rejections and denials, and factors that contributed to the length of time VA's TPAs have taken to pay providers. In addition, between April and June 2018, we interviewed a non-generalizable sample of 15 providers—including 7 that either currently participate or previously participated in the TriWest community provider network and 10 that either currently participate or previously participated in the Health Net community provider network—to identify any additional factors affecting payment time frames.[9] We selected the providers with the largest Choice Program claims volume from July 2017 through December 2017, based on the most recent TPA data available at the time we selected these providers.

To examine the actions taken by VA and the TPAs to reduce the length of time TPAs take to pay community providers for Choice Program claims, we reviewed VA and TPA documentation, such as contract modifications and policy documents. We also interviewed VA contracting officials and Office of Community Care officials as well as TPA officials. In addition, we interviewed the 15 selected providers to determine how claim payment timeliness issues have affected them. We assessed the actions taken by VA and the TPAs to

---

[8] In December 2016, VA issued an RFP for contractors to help administer its new Veterans Community Care Program.

[9] Tw o of these providers participated in both the TriWest and Health Net provider networks. The providers w e interviewed included hospital systems, group practices, and specialty providers, such as acupuncturists and chiropractors.

address the factors that contributed to the length of time taken to pay providers against federal standards for internal control for performing monitoring activities.[10]

We conducted this performance audit from February 2018 through September 2018 in accordance with generally accepted government auditing standards. Those standards require that we plan and perform our work to obtain sufficient, appropriate evidence to provide a reasonable basis for our findings and conclusions based on our audit objectives. We believe that the evidence obtained provides a reasonable basis for our findings and conclusions based on our audit objectives.

BACKGROUND

The Veterans Access, Choice, and Accountability Act of 2014 provided up to $10 billion in funding for veterans to obtain health care services from community providers through the Choice Program when veterans faced long wait times, lengthy travel distances, or other challenges accessing care at VA medical facilities.[11] The temporary authority and funding for the Choice Program was separate from other previously existing programs through which VA has the option to purchase care from community providers. Legislation enacted in August and December of 2017 and June 2018

---

[10] GAO, *Standards for Internal Control in the Federal Government*, GAO/AIMD-00-21.3.1 (Washington, D.C.: November 1999) and GAO-14-704G (Washington, D.C.: September 2014).Internal control is a process effected by an entity's oversight body, management, and other personnel that provides reasonable assurance that the objectives of an entity will be achieved.

[11] Pub. L. No. 113-146, §§ 101, 802, 128 Stat. 1754, 1755-1765, 1802-1803 (2014).

provided an additional \$9.4 billion for the Veterans Choice Fund.[12] Authority of the Choice Program will sunset on June 6, 2019.[13]

Responsibilities of the Choice Program TPAs

In October 2014, VA modified its existing contracts with two TPAs that were administering another VA community care program—the Patient-Centered Community Care program—to add certain administrative responsibilities associated with the Choice Program. For the Choice Program, each of the two TPAs—Health Net and TriWest—are responsible for managing networks of community providers who deliver care in a specific multi-state region. (See figure 1.) Specifically, the TPAs are responsible for establishing networks of community providers, scheduling appointments with community providers for eligible veterans, and paying community providers for their services.[14] Health Net's contract for administering the Choice Program will end on September 30, 2018, whereas TriWest will continue to administer the Choice Program until the program ends, which is expected to occur in fiscal year 2019.[15]

---

[12] VA Choice and Quality Employment Act of 2017, Pub. L. No. 115-46, § 101, 131 Stat. 958, 959 (Aug. 17, 2017) (providing an additional \$2.1 billion for the Veterans Choice Fund); Department of Homeland Security Blue Campaign Authorization Act of 2017, Pub. L. No. 115-96. Div. D, § 4001, 131 Stat. 2044, 2052-53 (Dec. 22, 2017) (providing an additional \$2.1 billion for the Veterans Choice Fund) and Pub. L. No. 115-182, tit. V, § 510, 132 Stat. 1392,__ (2018) (providing an additional \$5.2 billion for the Veterans Choice Fund).

[13] Pub. L. No. 115-182, tit. I, § 143, 132 Stat. 1393, __ (2018), amending section 101(p) of the Veterans Access, Choice, and Accountability Act of 2014, Pub. L. No. 113-146, 128 Stat. at 1763.

[14] Our previous w ork provides a detailed overview of VA's appointment scheduling process. See GAO, Veterans Choice Program: Improvements Needed to Address Access-Related Challenges as VA Plans Consolidation of Its Community Care Programs, GAO-18-281 (Washington, D.C.: June 4, 2018).

[15] In July 2018, Health Net began transitioning responsibilities for scheduling appointments to VA. However, Health Net will be responsible for processing claims and paying providers for care delivered prior to this date.

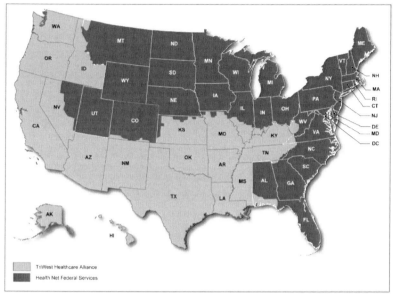

Source: GAO illustration based on Department of Veterans Affairs information (data);
Map Resources (map). | GAO-18-671.

Note: TriWest Healthcare Alliance is the TPA for American Samoa, Guam, and the Northern
Mariana Islands. Health Net Federal Services is the TPA for Puerto Rico and the U.S. Virgin
Islands.

Figure 1. Multi-state Regions Covered by the Veterans Choice Program's Third Party
Administrators (TPA).

Choice Program Claim Processing and Payment

VA's TPAs process claims they receive from community providers for
the care they deliver to veterans and pay providers for approved claims.
Figure 2 provides an overview of the steps the TPAs follow for processing
claims and paying community providers.

VA's contracts with the TPAs do not include a payment timeliness
requirement applicable to the payments TPAs make to community
providers. Instead, a contract modification effective in March 2016
established a non-enforceable "goal" of processing—approving, rejecting or
denying—and, if approved, paying clean claims within 30 days of receipt.

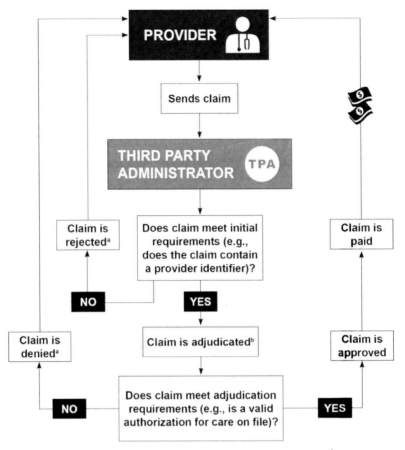

Source: GAO analysis of third party administrator (TPA) information | GAO-18-671.

[a] According to TPA officials, rejected claims are claims returned up front to providers due to, for example, the use of invalid claim forms and missing provider identification numbers. Denied claims are claims that contain the necessary data elements but do not pass required claim processing steps, which, for example, verify the veteran's eligibility for the Veterans Choice Program, that a valid authorization for care is on file, and that the claim is not a duplicate.

[b] Claim adjudication refers to the process of reviewing a claim and making the decision to approve or deny it. Claims being adjudicated are either classified as clean or non-clean claims. Clean claims are claims that contain all required data elements, while non-clean claims are those claims that are missing required data elements that the TPA must obtain before the claim is paid.

Figure 2. Steps TPAs Follow to Process and Pay Claims from Community Providers for Care Delivered Under the Veterans Choice Program.

To be reimbursed for its payments to providers, the TPAs in turn submit electronic invoices—or requests for payment—to VA. TPAs generate an invoice for every claim they receive from community providers and pay. VA reviews the TPAs' invoices and either approves or rejects them. Invoices may be rejected, for example, if care provided was not authorized. Approved invoices are paid, whereas rejected invoices are returned to the TPAs. The federal Prompt Payment Act requires VA to pay its TPAs within 30 days of receipt of invoices that it approves.[16]

VA's Planned Consolidated Community Care Program

The VA MISSION Act of 2018, among other things, requires VA to consolidate its community care programs once the Choice Program sunsets 1 year after the passage of the Act, authorizes VA to utilize a TPA for claims processing, and requires VA to reimburse community providers in a timely manner. Specifically, the act requires VA (or its TPAs) to pay community providers within 30 days of receipt for clean claims submitted electronically and within 45 days of receipt for clean claims submitted on paper.

In December 2016, prior to enactment of the VA MISSION Act of 2018, VA issued an RFP for contractors to help administer the Veterans Community Care Program. The Veterans Community Care Program will be similar to the current Choice Program in certain respects. For example, VA is planning to award community care network contracts to TPAs, which would establish regional networks of community providers and process and pay those providers' claims. However, unlike under the Choice Program, under the Veterans Community Care Program, VA is planning to have medical facilities—not the TPAs—generally be responsible for scheduling veterans' appointments with community providers.

---

[16] 31 U.S.C. § 3903(a)(1); 5 C.F.R. part 1315.

THE LENGTH OF TIME TAKEN BY TPAS TO PAY CLAIMS FROM COMMUNITY PROVIDERS HAS VARIED WIDELY, AND VA'S MONITORING OF THIS TIMELINESS HAS BEEN LIMITED

The Time TPAs Have Taken to Pay Claims Has Varied Widely, and Available Data Do Not Account for Payment Delays Due to Rejected or Denied Claims

From November 2014 through June 2018, VA's TPAs paid a total of about 16 million clean claims—which are claims that contain all required data elements—under the Choice Program, of which TriWest paid about 9.6 million claims and Health Net paid about 6.4 million. Data on the median number of days VA's TPAs have taken to pay clean claims each month show wide variation over the course of the Choice Program—from 7 days to 68 days. As discussed previously, in March 2016, VA established a non-enforceable goal for its TPAs to process and, if approved, pay clean claims within 30 days of receipt each month. Most recently, from January through June 2018, the median number of days taken to pay clean claims ranged from 26 to 28 days for TriWest, while it ranged from 28 to 44 days for Health Net. (See figure 3.)

In addition to the 16 million clean claims the TPAs paid from November 2014 through June 2018, during this time period they also paid approximately 650,000 claims (or 4 percent of all paid claims) that were classified as non-clean claims when first received after obtaining the required information. Non-clean claims are claims that are missing required information, which the TPA must obtain before the claim is paid. From November 2014 through June 2018, TriWest paid around 641,000 non-clean claims (or 6 percent of all paid claims) while Health Net paid about 9,600 non-clean claims (or less than 1 percent of all paid claims). Data on the median number of days VA's TPAs have taken to pay non-clean claims each month also show wide variation over the course of the Choice Program—from 9 days to 73 days. (See figure 4.)

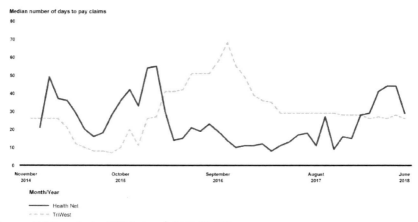

Source: GAO analysis of TPA data. | GAO-18-671.

Note: The Department of Veterans Affairs (VA) established a goal for its TPAs to process
and, if approved, pay clean claims within 30 calendar days of receipt. Clean claims are
claims that contain all required data elements. Health Net did not pay any clean claims
in November and December 2014 and TriWest did not pay any clean claims in
November 2014.

Figure 3. Median Number of Days to Pay Clean Claims through VA's Third Party
Administrators (TPA), November 2014 through June 2018.

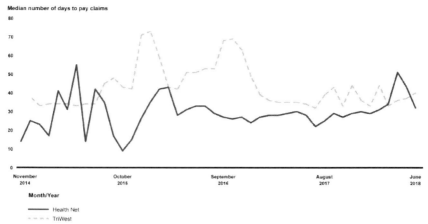

Source:GAO analysis of TPA data. | GAO-18-671.

Note: Non-clean claims are claims that are missing required data elements that the
Department of Veterans Affairs' (VA) TPA must obtain before the clam is paid. TriWest
did not pay any non-clean claims in November 2014.

Figure 4. Median Number of Days to Pay Non-Clean Claims through VA's Third Party
Administrators (TPA), November 2014 through June 2018.

The data on the time TPAs have taken to pay approved clean and non-clean claims do not fully account for the length of time taken to pay providers whose claims are initially rejected or denied, as, according to the TPAs, providers are generally required to submit a new claim when the original claim is rejected or denied.[17] Thus, providers that submit claims that are rejected or denied may experience a longer wait for payment for those claims or may not be paid at all. In some cases, providers' claims may be rejected or denied multiple times after resubmission.[18]

Stakeholders Identified Three Key Factors Affecting the Timeliness of Claim Payments to Community Providers under the Choice Program

VA and its TPAs identified three key factors affecting the timeliness of claim payments to community providers under the Choice Program: (1) VA's untimely payments of TPA invoices; (2) Choice Program contractual requirements related to provider reimbursement; and (3) inadequate provider education on filing Choice Program claims, as discussed below.

VA's Untimely Payments of TPA Invoices

According to VA and TPA officials, VA made untimely invoice payments to its TPAs—that is, payments made more than 30 days from the date VA received the TPAs' invoices—which resulted in the TPAs at times having insufficient funds available to pay community providers under the Choice Program.[19] A VA Office of Inspector General (OIG) report estimated

---

[17] According to TPA officials, rejected claims are claims returned up front to providers due to, for example, the use of invalid claim forms and missing provider identification numbers. Denied claims are claims that contain the necessary data elements but do not pass required claim processing steps, which, for example, verify the veteran's eligibility for the Choice Program, that a valid authorization for care is on file, and that the claim is not a duplicate.

[18] From November 2014 through June 2018, Health Net's data show that it denied about 29 percent of all claims community providers submitted to the Choice Program, with the denial rate having varied from month to month.

[19] TriWest officials attributed payment delays to VA's process for re-adjudicating community provider claims as part of its review of TPA invoices. This process resulted in invoice rejections, which the TPAs subsequently appealed. We cannot quantify the extent to which

that from November 2014 through September 2016, 50 percent of VA's payments to its TPAs during this time frame were untimely.[20] VA officials stated that VA's untimely payments to the TPAs resulted from limitations in its fee-basis claims system, which VA used at the beginning of the Choice Program to process all TPA invoices.[21] In addition, the VA OIG found that VA underestimated the number of staff necessary to process Choice Program invoices in a timely manner.

Choice Program Reimbursement Requirements

According to VA and TPA officials, three Choice Program requirements, some of which were more stringent than similar requirements in other federal health care programs, led to claim denials, which, in turn, contributed to the length of time TPAs have taken to pay community providers when the providers did not meet these requirements:

1. Medical documentation requirement. Prior to a March 2016 contract modification, VA required providers to submit relevant medical documentation with their claims as a condition of payment from the TPAs.[22] According to TriWest officials, those Choice Program claims that did not include medical documentation were classified by TriWest as non-clean claims and placed in pending status until the documentation was received. When community providers did not provide the supporting medical documentation after a certain

---

VA's untimely payments to the TPAs affected the length of time the TPAs' took to pay providers because w e are unable to examine the impact of this factor in isolation from other factors impacting the time the TPAs took to pay providers.

[20] See Department of Veterans Affairs, Office of Inspector General, *Veterans Health Administration: Audit of the Timeliness and Accuracy of Choice Payments Processed Through the Fee Basis Claims System,* Report No. 15-03036-47 (Washington, D.C.: Dec. 12, 2017). VA's OIG reviewed a sample of 646 paid claims for the tw o TPAs from November 1, 2014 through September 30, 2016.

[21] The fee-basis claims system was used nationwide by VA to process TPA invoices. After the TPAs adjudicated and paid community provider claims, they submitted invoices to VA. VA then used the fee basis claims system to re-adjudicate the original claim and determine w hether the TPA's invoice for the claim should be paid.

[22] Medicare and TRICARE, the Department of Defense's health care program, generally do not require providers to submit medical documentation as a condition of claim payment. See GAO-16-353.

period of time, TriWest typically denied their claims. According to Health Net officials, Choice Program claims that did not include medical documentation were denied by Health Net.

2. Timely filing requirement. VA requires providers to file Choice Program claims within 180 business days from the end of an episode of care.[23] TPAs deny claims that are not filed within the required time frame.

3. Authorization requirement. VA requires authorizations for community providers to serve veterans under the Choice Program and receive reimbursement for their services; however, if community providers deliver care after an authorization period or include services that are not authorized, the TPAs typically deny their claims.[24] According to TPA data, denials related to authorizations are among the most common reasons the TPAs deny community provider claims.

Inadequate Provider Education on Filing Choice Program Claims

According to VA and TPA officials as well as providers we interviewed, issues related to inadequate provider education may have contributed to the length of time it has taken the TPAs to pay community providers under the Choice Program. These issues have included providers submitting claims with errors, submitting claims to the wrong payer, or otherwise failing to meet Choice Program requirements. For example, some VA community care programs require the claims to be sent to one of VA's claims processing locations, while the Choice Program requires claims to be sent to TriWest or Health Net. Claims sent to the wrong entity are rejected or denied and have to be resubmitted to the correct payer. Ten of the 15 providers we interviewed stated that that they lacked education and/or training on the

---

[23] Health Net's agreement with its community providers requires the submission of Choice Program claims within 120 business days of the date of service.

[24] VA officials stated that authorization-related claim denials can occur for many reasons, including the provider delivering care that was not listed on the authorization and the authorization being expired, which can occur if a veteran cancelled the original appointment and rescheduled the appointment outside of the authorization's validity period. In contrast to the Choice Program, Medicare typically does not require authorizations for beneficiaries to obtain care and TRICARE only requires authorizations for certain types of care.

claims filing process when they first began participating in the Choice Program, including knowing where to file claims and the documentation needed to file claims that would be processed successfully. Four of these 10 providers stated that they learned how to submit claims through trial and error.

VA's Monitoring of Claim Payment Timeliness Has Been Limited under the Choice Program, but VA Plans to Strengthen Monitoring under the Veterans Community Care Program

At the infancy of the Choice Program, November 2014 through March 2016, VA was unable to monitor the timeliness of its TPAs' payments to community providers because it did not require the TPAs to provide data on the length of time taken to pay these claims. Effective in March 2016, VA modified its TPA contracts and subsequently began monitoring TPA payment timeliness, requiring TPAs to report information on claims processing and payment timeliness as well as information on claim rejections and denials. However, because VA had not established a payment timeliness requirement, VA officials said that VA had limited ability to penalize TPAs or compel them to take corrective actions to address untimely claim payments to community providers. Instead, the March 2016 contract modification established a non-enforceable goal for the TPAs to process and pay clean claims within 30 days of receipt. As of July 2018, according to VA officials, VA did not have a contractual requirement it could use to help ensure that community providers received timely payments in the Choice Program.

Officials from VA's Office of Community Care told us that VA's experience with payment timeliness in the Choice Program informed VA's RFP for new contracts for the Veterans Community Care Program, which includes provisions that strengthen VA's ability to monitor its future TPAs. For example, in addition to requiring future TPAs to submit weekly reports on claim payment timeliness as well as claim rejections and denials, VA's RFP includes claim payment timeliness standards that are similar to those in the Department of

Defense's TRICARE program.[25] Specifically, according to the RFP, TPAs in the Veterans Community Care Program will be required to

- process and pay, if approved, 98 percent of clean claims within 30 days of receipt,
- return claims, other than clean claims, to the provider with a clear explanation of deficiencies within 30 days of original receipt, and
- process resubmitted claims within 30 days of resubmission receipt.[26]

The RFP also identifies monitoring techniques that VA may employ to assess compliance with these requirements, including periodic inspections and audits. VA officials told us that VA will develop a plan for monitoring the TPAs' performance on these requirements once the contracts are awarded.

VA HAS ADDRESSED SOME BUT NOT ALL OF THE KEY FACTORS AFFECTING THE TIMELINESS OF CLAIM PAYMENTS TO COMMUNITY PROVIDERS UNDER THE CHOICE PROGRAM

We found that VA has made system and process changes that improved its ability to pay TPA invoices in a timely manner. However, while VA has modified two Choice Program requirements that contributed to provider claim payment delays, it has not fully addressed delays associated with authorizations for care. Furthermore, while VA and its TPAs have taken

---

[25] TRICARE is the Department of Defense's healthcare program.

[26] Some of the claim payment timeliness standards in VA's RFP differ from the requirements set forth in the VA MISSION Act of 2018. For example, the act requires VA (or its TPAs) to pay providers within 30 days for claims submitted electronically and within 45 days for claims submitted on paper, whereas the RFP does not differentiate between claims filed electronically or on paper. VA officials told us that they have not determined how to reconcile the differences in the payment timeliness standards.

steps to educate community providers in order to help prevent claims processing issues, 9 of the 15 providers we interviewed reported poor customer service when attempting to resolve these issues.

VA Has Changed Its System and Processes for Paying TPA Invoices in Order to Improve Its Ability to Pay TPAs in a Timely Manner

VA has taken steps to reduce untimely payments to its TPAs, which contributed to delayed TPA payments to providers, by implementing a new system and updating its processes for paying TPA invoices so that it can pay these invoices more quickly. Specifically, VA has made the following changes:

- In March 2016, VA negotiated a contract modification with both TPAs that facilitated the processing of certain TPA invoices outside of the fee basis claims system from March 2016 through July 2016.[27] According to VA officials, due to the increasing volume of invoices that the TPAs were expecting to submit to VA during this time period, without this process change, VA would have experienced a high volume of TPA invoices entering its fee basis claims system, which could have exacerbated payment timeliness issues.
- In February through April 2017, VA transitioned all TPA invoice payments from its fee basis claims system to an expedited payment

---

[27] Effective in March 2016, VA decoupled, or removed, the requirement that medical documentation be submitted to the TPA as a condition of claims payment (this contract modification is discussed later in this report). VA allowed the invoices from these "decoupled" claims to be processed outside of the fee basis claims system, while non-decoupled claims continued to be processed through the fee basis claims system. In addition, VA executed contract modifications with Health Net in October 2016 and TriWest in November 2016 that issued lump-sum payments to the TPAs to address backlogged Choice Program claims. The VA OIG examined the accuracy of VA's lump-sum payments in a report issued in September 2018. See Department of Veterans Affairs, Office of Inspector General, *Veterans Health Administration: Bulk Payments Made under Patient-Centered Community Care/Veterans Choice Program Contracts,* Report No. 17-02713- 231 (Washington, D.C.: Sept. 6, 2018).

process under a new system called Plexis Claims Manager.[28] VA officials told us that instead of re-adjudicating community provider claims as part of its review of TPA invoices, Plexis Claims Manager performed up front checks in order to pay invoices more quickly, and any differences in billed and paid amounts were addressed after payments were issued to the TPAs.

- In January 2018, VA transitioned to a newer version of the Plexis Claims Manager that enabled VA to once again re-adjudicate community provider claims as part of processing TPA invoices, but in a timelier manner compared with the fee basis claims system. According to VA officials, this is due to the automation of claims processing under Plexis Claims Manager, which significantly reduced the need for manual claims processing by VA staff that occurred under the fee basis claims system. Based on VA data, as of July 2018, VA is paying 92 percent of TriWest's submitted invoices within 7 days, with payments being made in an average of 4 days, and 90 percent of Health Net's invoices within 7 days, with payments being made in an average of 4 days under the newer version of Plexis Claims Manager.[29]

In addition to steps taken to address untimely payments to the TPAs under the current Choice Program contracts, VA has taken steps to help assure payment timeliness in the forthcoming Veterans Community Care Program. Specifically, the RFP includes a requirement for VA to reimburse TPAs within 14 days of receiving an invoice. VA officials stated that to achieve this metric, they are implementing a new payment system that will replace Plexis Claims Manager and will no longer re-adjudicate TPA invoices prior to payment.

---

[28] This transition occurred for TriWest invoices in February 2017 and for Health Net invoices in April 2017.

[29] According to VA officials, payments to TriWest are faster as the invoices TriWest submits typically contain fewer errors than Health Net's invoices. We did not examine the validity or accuracy of VA's statistics.

VA Has Modified Two Choice Program Requirements That Contributed to Provider Payment Delays, but Has Not Fully Addressed Delays Associated with Authorizations for Care

VA has issued a contract modification and waivers for two Choice Program contract requirements that contributed to provider payment delays—(1) the medical documentation requirement and (2) the timely filing requirement. However, while VA issued a contract modification to amend the requirements for obtaining authorizations for Choice Program care, provider payment delays associated with requesting these authorizations may persist, because VA is not ensuring that VA medical centers review and approve these requests within required time frames.

Elimination of Medical Documentation Requirement

Effective beginning March 2016, VA issued a contract modification that eliminated the requirement that community providers must submit medical documentation as a condition of receiving payment for their claims. Data from one TPA showed a reduction in non-clean claims following the implementation of this contract modification.[30] For example, starting in April 2016, after this modification was executed, almost 100 percent of claims submitted to TriWest were classified as clean claims, as opposed to 49 percent of claims submitted in March 2016. However, when the modification first went into effect in March 2016, TriWest and Health Net officials stated that they processed a large amount of claims from community providers that had previously been pended or denied because they lacked medical documentation and, in turn, submitted a large number of invoices to VA for reimbursement. As previously discussed, to help address the increased number of TPA invoices, VA issued lump-sum payments to the TPAs during this time period.

---

[30] Data from Health Net did not show a reduction in non-clean claims, as Health Net officials told us that claims that were missing medical documentation prior to the implementation of this contract modification were denied.

Modification of Timely Filing Requirement

In February and May 2018, VA issued waivers that gave TPAs the authority to allow providers to resubmit rejected or denied claims more than 180 days after the end of the episode of care if the original claims were submitted timely—that is, within 180 days of the end of the episode of care. VA officials stated that the waivers were intended to reduce the number of rejected and denied claims by giving community providers the ability to resubmit previously rejected or denied claims for which the date of service occurred more than 180 days ago. VA's waivers were implemented as follows:

- In February 2018, VA issued a waiver that allowed community providers to resubmit certain claims rejected or denied for specific reasons when the provider or TPA could verify that the provider made an effort to submit the claim prior to the claims submission deadline.[31]
- In May 2018, VA issued a second waiver that removed the 180 day timeliness requirement for all Choice Program claims. The waiver also provided instructions to the TPAs on informing providers that they may resubmit claims rejected or denied for specific reasons and how the TPAs are to process the resubmitted claims.[32]

In regards to the first waiver, TPA officials stated that the processing of those resubmitted claims adversely affected the timeliness of the TPAs' payments to community providers because the waiver resulted in a large influx of older claims. As the second waiver was in the process of being implemented by the two TPAs at the time we conducted our work, we were unable to determine if the second waiver affected the TPAs' provider payment timeliness.

---

[31] Some specific reasons for resubmission listed in the w aiver include, but are not limited to, paper claims rejected by the TPA due to scanning issues or coding errors.

[32] Some specific reasons for resubmission listed in the w aiver include, but are not limited to, paper claims rejected by the TPA due to scanning issues or claims incorrectly submitted by the provider to the incorrect payer (for example, Choice Program claims sent to VA directly instead of the TPA).

Changes to Authorization of Care Requirement

VA issued a contract modification in January 2017 to expand the time period for which authorizations for community providers to provide care to veterans under the Choice Program are valid.[33] In addition, in May 2017, VA expanded the scope of the services covered by authorizations, allowing them to encompass an overall course of treatment, rather than a specific service or set of services.[34] According to VA officials, the changes VA made related to the authorization of care requirement were also intended to reduce the need for secondary authorization requests (SAR). Community providers request SARs when veterans need health care services that exceed the period or scope of the original authorizations. Community providers are required to submit SARs to their TPA, which, in turn, submits the SARs to the authorizing VA medical facility for review and approval. Both Health Net and TriWest officials told us that since VA changed the time frame and scope of authorizations, the number of SARs has decreased.

Despite efforts to decrease the number of SARs, payment delays or claim denials are likely to continue if SARs are needed. We found that VA is not ensuring that VA medical facilities are reviewing and approving SARs within required time frames. VA policy states that VA medical facilities are to review and make SAR approval decisions within 5 business days of receipt.[35] However, officials from one of the TPAs and 7 of the 15 providers we interviewed stated that VA medical facilities are not reviewing and approving SARs in a timely manner. According to TriWest officials, as of May 2018, VA medical facilities in their regions were taking an average of 11 days to review and make approval decisions on SARs, with four facilities taking over 30 days for this process.

According to an official from VA's Office of Community Care, VA does not currently collect reliable national data to track the extent of nonadherence to the VA policy to review and make SAR approval decisions

---

[33] Specifically, the modification extended the validity period of each authorization to 7 days prior to the authorization start date and 60 days after the authorization end date.

[34] For example, a veteran who requires joint replacement surgery can be expected to receive physical therapy as part of that treatment. With bundled services outlined in the authorization, physical therapy would be covered without the need for an additional authorization.

[35] See VA Secondary Authorization Request Escalation Guidelines Standard Operating Procedure (Sept. 27, 2016).

within 5 business days. The official told us that instead, VA relies on employees assigned to each Veterans Integrated Service Network to monitor data on VA medical facilities' timeliness in making these SAR approval decisions.[36] If a VA medical facility is found not to be in adherence with the SAR policy, the official told us that staff assigned to the Veterans Integrated Service Network attempt to identify the reasons for nonadherence, and perform certain corrective actions, including providing education to the facility.[37] Despite these actions, the official told us that there are still VA medical facilities not in adherence with VA's SAR approval policy.

According to a VA official, VA is in the process of piloting software for managing authorizations that will allow VA to better track SAR approval time frames across VA medical facilities in the future. However, even after this planned software is implemented, if VA does not use the data to monitor and assess SAR approval decision time frames VA will be unable to ensure that all VA medical facilities are adhering to the policy. Standards for internal control in the Federal Government state that management should establish and operate monitoring activities to evaluate whether a specific function or process is operating effectively and take corrective actions as necessary. Furthermore, monitoring such data will allow VA to identify and take actions as needed to address any identified challenges VA medical facilities are encountering in meeting the required approval decision time frames. Without monitoring data to ensure that all VA medical facilities are adhering to the SAR approval time frames as outlined in VA policy, community providers may delay care until the SARs are approved or provide care without SAR approval. This in turn increases the likelihood that the community providers' claims will be denied. Further, continued nonadherence to VA's SAR policy raises concerns about VA's ability to ensure timely approval of SARs when VA medical facilities

---

[36] The official told us that data on SAR approval time frames are limited as the system that collects this information was not originally intended to be used to report that type of data. VA's health care system is divided into 18 health care networks, referred to as Veterans Integrated Service Networks, which are responsible for managing and overseeing VA medical facilities within a defined geographic area.

[37] According to the official, reasons for nonadherence could include a lack of staff and facilities not using time-saving tools VA has made available to them. We have previously identified inadequate staffing at VA medical facilities as a factor that impacts access to care through the Choice Program. See GAO-18-281.

assume more responsibilities for ensuring veterans' access to care under the forthcoming Veterans Community Care Program.

TPAs Have Taken Steps to Improve Provider Education to Help Providers Resolve Claims Processing Issues, but Many Providers Still Report Poor Customer Service

We found that VA and its TPAs have taken steps to educate community providers in order to help prevent claims processing issues that have contributed to the length of time TPAs have taken to pay these providers. Despite these efforts, 9 of the 15 providers we interviewed reported poor customer service when attempting to resolve claims payment issues.

While VA's contracts with the TPAs do not include requirements for educating and training providers on the Choice Program, both TPAs have taken steps to educate community providers on how to successfully submit claims under the Choice Program. Specifically, TriWest and Health Net officials told us that they have taken various steps to educate community providers on submitting claims correctly, including sending monthly newsletters, emails, and faxes to communicate changes to the Choice Program; updating their websites with claims processing information; and holding meetings with some providers monthly or quarterly to resolve claims processing issues. Officials from both TPAs also told us that they provided one-on-one training to some providers on the claims submission process to help reduce errors when submitting claims. In addition, VA's RFP for the Veterans Community Care Program contracts includes requirements to provide an annual training program curriculum and an initial on-boarding and ongoing outreach and education program for community providers, which includes training on the claims submission and payment processes and TPA points of contact.

VA and the TPAs have also made efforts to help providers resolve claims processing issues and outstanding payments. For example,

- VA launched its "top 20 provider initiative" in January 2018 to work directly with community providers with high dollar amounts of unpaid claims and resolve ongoing claims payment issues. This initiative included creating rapid response teams to work with community providers to settle unpaid claim balances within 90 days and working with both TPAs to increase the number of clean claims paid in less than 30 days. In addition, VA has developed webinars on VA's community care programs and—in conjunction with trade organizations and health care systems—has delivered provider education on filing claims properly.
- TriWest officials stated that it has educated the customer service staff at its claims processing sub-contractor, who field community provider calls regarding claims processing issues, to help ensure that the staff are familiar with Choice Program changes and can effectively assist community providers and resolve claims processing issues. Internal TriWest data show that providers' average wait time to speak to a customer service representative about claims processing issues decreased from as high as 18 minutes in 2016 to as low as 2.5 minutes in 2018.
- Health Net officials were unable to provide data, but stated that since the fourth quarter of 2017, Health Net has decreased the time it takes for a community provider to speak with a customer service representative by adding additional staff and extending the hours in which providers can call with questions. In addition, Health Net officials stated that they have required customer service staff to undergo additional training related to resolving claims processing issues.

Despite these efforts, 7 of the 10 providers that participate in the Health Net network and 2 of the 7 providers that participate in the TriWest network we interviewed between April and June 2018 told us that when they contact the TPAs' customer service staff to address claim processing questions, such as how to resolve claim rejections or denials, they experience lengthy hold times, sometimes exceeding one hour. In addition, 7 of the 15 providers we spoke with told us they typically reach employees who are unable to answer their questions. According to these providers, this experience frustrated them, as they often did not understand why a claim had been denied or rejected, and they required assistance correcting the claim so it could be resubmitted. One community provider stated that their common practice to resolve questions or concerns was to call customer service enough times until they received the same answer twice from a TPA representative. In addition, 5 of the 10 Health Net providers we interviewed stated that they have significant outstanding claim balances owed to them. One of these providers—who reported over $3 million in outstanding claims—stressed the importance of being able to effectively resolve claims issues with TPA customer service staff, as the administrative burden of following up on outstanding claim balances takes time away from caring for patients.

The issues concerning customer service wait times and TPA staff inability to resolve some claims processing issues reported by community providers appear to be inconsistent with VA contractual requirements.

VA's current Choice Program contracts require the TPAs to establish a customer call center to respond to calls from veterans and non-VA providers. The contract requires specified levels of service for telephone inquiries at the call center. For example, VA requires TPA representatives to answer customer service calls within an average speed of 30 seconds or less and requires 85 percent of all inquiries to be fully and completely answered during the initial telephone call. However, VA officials explained that VA does not enforce the contractual requirement for responding to calls from community providers. Furthermore, according to these officials, VA allows the TPAs to prioritize calls from veterans. Officials from VA's Office of General Counsel, Procurement Law Group, confirmed that this requirement does apply to the TPAs' handling of calls from community providers. Because VA does not enforce the customer service requirement for providers, VA has not collected data on or monitored the TPAs' compliance with these requirements for providers' calls.

As previously stated, standards for internal control in the Federal Government state that management should establish and operate monitoring activities to evaluate whether a specific function or process is operating effectively and take corrective actions as necessary. Without collecting data and monitoring customer service requirements for provider calls, VA does not have information on the extent to which community providers face challenges when contacting the TPAs about claims payment issues that could contribute to the amount of time it takes to successfully file claims and receive reimbursement for services under the Choice Program. This, in turn, poses a risk to the Choice Program to the extent that community providers who face these challenges decide not to serve veterans under the Choice Program.

Looking forward, VA has included customer service requirements in its RFP for the Veterans Community Care Program contracts, and VA officials have told us that these requirements are applicable to provider calls. For example, the RFP includes a requirement for its future TPAs to establish and maintain call centers to address inquiries from community providers and has established customer service performance metrics to monitor call center performance.[38] Monitoring data on provider calls under the contracts will be important as Veterans Community Care Program TPAs will continue to be responsible for building provider networks, processing claims, and resolving claims processing issues.

CONCLUSION

The Choice Program relies on community providers to deliver care to eligible veterans when VA is unable to provide timely and accessible care at

---

[38] The RFP also includes a requirement for future TPAs to conduct community provider satisfaction surveys.

its own facilities. Although VA has taken steps to improve the timeliness of TPA claim payments to providers, VA is not collecting data or monitoring compliance with two Choice Program requirements, and this could adversely affect the timeliness with which community providers are paid under the Choice Program. First, VA does not have complete data allowing it to effectively monitor adherence with its policy for VA medical facilities to review SARs within 5 days of receipt, which impacts its ability to meet the requirement. To the extent that VA medical facilities delay these reviews and approvals, community providers may have to delay care or deliver care that is not authorized, which in turn increases the likelihood that the providers' claims will be denied and the providers will not be paid. Second, VA requires the TPAs to establish a customer call center to respond to calls from veterans and non-VA providers. However, VA does not enforce the contractual requirement for responding to calls from community providers and allows the TPAs to prioritize calls from veterans. Consequently, VA is not collecting data, monitoring, or enforcing compliance with its contractual requirements for the TPAs to provide timely customer service to providers. As a result, VA does not have information on the extent to which community providers face challenges when contacting the TPAs about claims payment issues, which could contribute to the amount of time it takes to receive reimbursement for services.

To the extent that these issues make community providers less willing to continue participating in the Choice Program and the forthcoming Veterans Community Care Program, they pose a risk to VA's ability to successfully implement these programs and ensure veterans' timely access to care.

RECOMMENDATIONS FOR EXECUTIVE ACTION

We are making the following two recommendations to VA:

Once VA's new software for managing authorizations has been fully implemented, the Undersecretary for Health should monitor data on SAR approval decision time frames to ensure VA medical facilities are in adherence with VA policy, assess the reasons for nonadherence with the policy, and take corrective actions as necessary. (Recommendation 1)

The Undersecretary for Health should collect data and monitor compliance with the Choice Program contractual requirements pertaining to customer service for community providers, and take corrective actions as necessary. (Recommendation 2)

AGENCY COMMENTS

We provided a draft of this report to VA for review and comment. In its written comments, reproduced in appendix I, VA concurred with our two recommendations and said it is taking steps to address them. For example, VA plans to implement software in spring 2019 that will automate the SAR process and allow for streamlined reporting and monitoring of SAR timeliness to ensure ongoing compliance. Additionally, VA has included provider customer service performance requirements and metrics in its Veterans Community Care Program RFP, and will require future contractors to provide a monthly report to VA on their call center operations and will implement quarterly provider satisfaction surveys.

We are sending copies of this report to the Secretary of Veterans Affairs, the Under Secretary for Health, appropriate congressional committees, and other interested parties. This report is also available at no charge on the GAO Web site at http://www.gao.gov.

Sincerely yours,

Sharon M. Silas
Acting Director, Health Care

APPENDIX I: COMMENTS FROM THE DEPARTMENT OF VETERANS AFFAIRS

THE SECRETARY OF VETERANS AFFAIRS
WASHINGTON
September 13, 2018

Ms. Sharon Silas
Acting Director
Health Care
U.S. Government Accountability Office
441 G Street, NW
Washington, DC 20548

Dear Ms. Silas:

The Department of Veterans Affairs (VA) has reviewed the Government Accountability Office (GAO) draft report: *"VETERANS CHOICE PROGRAM: Further Improvements Needed to Help Ensure Timely Payments to Community Providers"* (GAO-18-671).

The enclosure sets forth the actions to be taken to address the GAO draft report recommendations.

VA appreciates the opportunity to comment on your draft report.

Sincerely,

Robert L. Wilkie

Enclosure

Department of Veterans Affairs (VA) Comments to
Government Accountability Office (GAO) Draft Report
**"VETERANS CHOICE PROGRAM: Further Improvements Needed to Help
Ensure Timely Payments to Community Providers"**
(GAO-18-671)

Recommendation 1: Once VA's new software for managing authorizations has
been fully implemented, the Undersecretary for Health should monitor data on
SAR approval decision timeframes to ensure VA medical facilities are in
adherence with VA policy, assess the reasons for nonadherence with the policy,
and take corrective actions as necessary.

VA Comment: Concur. The Department of Veterans Affairs (VA) Office of Community
Care (OCC) has been monitoring secondary authorization requests (SAR) timeliness via
weekly manual data extractions since March 2016. The current timeframe for SAR
adjudication is 5 days. In September 2017, OCC began monitoring SAR timeliness via
the OCC Top 8 Metrics report, a report that highlights key performance metrics
important to Veterans Integrated Service Network (VISN)/VA medical center (VAMC)
community care activities. OCC has trended data from the Top 8 metrics report since
September 2017 and has used this information to identify and offer proactive assistance
to low performing sites. Weekly calls between OCC Field Support staff, VISN/VAMC
Business Implementation Managers, and station leadership have been held to support
the lowest performing VISNs. The calls have been used to identify and assess
barriers/challenges, agree upon improvement actions, and to provide additional training
and tips on process/tool usage to resolve underperformance. As of July 2018, the total
number of SARs pending 5 days or greater has been reduced by 56 percent to 22,789
down from 51,985 when monitoring via the Top 8 Metrics report began.

Health Share Referral Manager (HSRM) Version 5, will automate SAR reporting and
tracking to allow for streamlined reporting and monitoring of their timeliness. HSRM is a
web-based software platform that streamlines the community care referral and
authorization process and improves information-sharing between VA and community
providers. Critically, HSRM addresses issues with our current referral and authorization
business processes that require extensive manual procedures and re-entry of data
across disparate systems.

HSRM Version 5 will be released in May 2019, and OCC will utilize its capability to
continue leading monitoring efforts to ensure compliance. HSRM is currently being
tested at three sites, and implementation across all of the Veterans Health
Administration is planned for the Spring 2019. This automation will equip OCC and
VISN/VAMC leadership with real-time access to SAR timeliness data to ensure ongoing
monitoring and compliance. OCC will continue to work with VISN/VAMC Business
Implementation Managers and station leadership to identify barriers and actions for
improvement as outliers are noted in the new automated reports. The status is in
process with a target completion date of June 2019.

Department of Veterans Affairs (VA) Comments to
Government Accountability Office (GAO) Draft Report
*"VETERANS CHOICE PROGRAM: Further Improvements Needed to Help
Ensure Timely Payments to Community Providers"*
(GAO-18-671)

Recommendation 2: The Under Secretary for Health should collect data and
monitor compliance with the Choice Program contractual requirements pertaining
to customer service for community providers, and take corrective actions as
necessary.

VA Comment: Concur. VA does not currently have the ability to monitor and assess
the performance of customer service operations included in the current Veterans Choice
Program (VCP) contracts. The VCP Performance Work Statement (PWS) Section 3(c)
includes only a contractual requirement for the Third-Party Administrator (TPA) to
establish a call center to provide customer service for community providers and
provides guidance for its operations. However, there are no Quality Assurance
Surveillance Plans, related to performance monitoring of these operations, nor any
mechanisms for the VA to collect data and monitor compliance with the limited VCP
contractual requirements.

Moving forward, VA elected to implement call center handling best practices and has
included additional requirements for Customer Service in the Community Care Network
(CCN) Request for Proposals (RFP). Section 6.2 of the RFP includes requirements for
toll-free telephone lines, access to a Real Time Chat function, and automated phone
call back to respond to online and telephonic inquiries, and seeks to ensure coverage
across a variety of inquiry categories including: status of referrals, prior authorization
status, claims status and issues, and complaints.

Section 6.8 of the CCN RFP further details the Call Center Operations and Customer
Service Technology Performance Requirements and Metrics. The contractor's
customer service capabilities must meet the performance standards as defined below.

Provider Inquiry Call Center Handling Standards

Metric	Performance Rate
Blockage Rate	less than 5 percent
Call Abandonment Rates	5 percent or less
Average Speed of Answer	30 Seconds or less
First Call Resolution	85 percent or higher
Response Accuracy	90 percent or higher
Real-Time Chat Satisfaction	90 percent or higher

The contractor must provide a monthly report on their call center operations
summarizing call center inquiries, performance metrics, open issues, and trends. In
addition, Section 6.7 of the CCN RFP provides that the TPA will be required to submit a

Department of Veterans Affairs (VA) Comments to
Government Accountability Office (GAO) Draft Report
***"VETERANS CHOICE PROGRAM: Further Improvements Needed to Help
Ensure Timely Payments to Community Providers"***
(GAO-18-671)

quarterly provider satisfaction survey report of all community providers who submitted claims that quarter. The contractor must report to VA the results of such surveys 60 days following conclusion of the survey quarter. The data provided in the quarterly reports and in the quarterly face to face Performance Management Reviews shall be used to review performance, identify emerging issues and address current issues, and maintain an effective customer service relationship between the contractor and VA. The status is in process with a target completion date of December 2019.

INDEX

N

O

P

R

W

Adaptive Sports and Paralympic Grant Programs for Veterans: Overview, Breakdowns and Assessments

EDITOR: Devin Morales

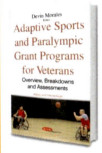

SERIES: Military and Veteran Issues

BOOK DESCRIPTION: This book reviews how VA selected grantees to provide activities for veterans and service members with disabilities; how VA monitors grantees' use of funds; and what programs and activities were supported with fiscal year 2014 funds, and what is known about its benefits.

SOFTCOVER ISBN: 978-1-63484-916-6
RETAIL PRICE: $62

Veterans: Political, Social and Health Issues

EDITOR: Milton Townsend

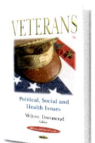

SERIES: Military and Veteran Issues

BOOK DESCRIPTION: This book provides insights into the political, social and health issues for Veterans in today's society.

HARDCOVER ISBN: 978-1-63484-691-2
RETAIL PRICE: $160